The Eradication of Infectious Diseases

Goal of this Dahlem Workshop:

To identify the biological/epidemiological, cost/benefit, and societal/political criteria for eradication of infectious diseases.

Dahlem Workshop Report

Held and published on behalf of the
Freie Universität Berlin

Sponsored by:
Deutsche Forschungsgemeinschaft

The Eradication of Infectious Diseases

Edited by

W.R. DOWDLE and D.R. HOPKINS

Report of the Dahlem Workshop on
The Eradication of Infectious Diseases
Berlin, March 16–22, 1997

Program Advisory Committee:
W.R. Dowdle and D.R. Hopkins, Chairpersons
R.A. Goodman, A.J. Hall, and B. Schwartländer

JOHN WILEY & SONS
Chichester • New York • Weinheim • Brisbane • Singapore • Toronto

Other Wiley Editorial Offices

John Wiley & Sons, Inc. 605 Third Avenue,
New York, NY 10158–0012, U.S.A.

VCH Verlagsgesellschaft mbH, Pappelallee 3,
D–69469 Weinheim, Germany

Jacaranda Wiley Ltd., 33 Part Road, Milton,
Queensland 4064, Australia

John Wiley & Sons (Asia) Pte Ltd., 2 Clementi Loop #02–01,
Jin Xing Distripark, Singapore 129809

John Wiley & Sons (Canada) Ltd., 22 Worcester Road,
Rexdale, Ontario M9W 1L1, Canada

Library of Congress Cataloging-in-Publication Data
Dahlem Workshop on The Eradication of Infectious Diseases (1997:
  Berlin, Germany)
    The eradication of infectious diseases: report of the Dahlem
  Workshop on The Eradication of Infectious Diseases. Berlin. March
  16–22, 1997. / edited by W.R. Dowdle and D.R. Hopkins.
      p. cm. — (Dahlem workshop reports)
    "Program advisory committee: W.R. Dowdle and D.R. Hopkins, chairpersons,
  R.A. Goodman, A.J. Hall, and B. Schwartländer."
    Includes bibliographical references and index.
    ISBN 0–471–98089–7 (alk. paper)
    1. Communicable diseases — Prevention — Congresses. I. Dowdle,
  Walter R. II. Hopkins, Donald R. 1934– . III. Series.
  RA643.D34 1997   97–41829
  614.4'4—dc21   CIP

British Library Cataloging-in-Publication Data
A catalog record for this book is available from the British Library

ISBN   0 471 980897

Editorial Staff of Dahlem Konferenzen: J. Lupp, C. Rued-Engel, G. Custance
Typeset in 10/12 pt Times by Dahlem Konferenzen

Printed and bound in Great Britain by Biddles Ltd., Guildford, Surrey.

This book is printed on acid-free paper responsibly manufactured from sustainable forestation,
for which at least two trees are planted for each one used for paper production.

Contents

The Dahlem Konferenzen

In 1974, the Stifterverband für die Deutsche Wissenschaft[1] in cooperation with the Deutsche Forschungsgemeinschaft[2] founded the *Dahlem Konferenzen*. It was created to promote an interdisciplinary exchange of scientific ideas as well as to stimulate cooperation in research among international scientists. Dahlem Konferenzen proved itself to be an invaluable tool for communication in science, and so, to secure its long-term future, it was integrated into the Freie Universität Berlin in January, 1990.

As has been evident over recent years, scientific research has become highly interdisciplinary. Now, before real progress can be made in any one field, the concepts, methods, and strategies of related fields must be understood and able to be applied. Coordinated research efforts, scientific cooperation, and basic communication between the disciplines and the scientists themselves must be promoted in order for science to advance.

To meet these demands, Dahlem Konferenzen created a special type of forum for communication, now internationally recognized as the *Dahlem Workshop Model*. These workshops are the framework in which coherent discussions between the disciplines take place and are focused around a topic of high priority interest to the disciplines concerned. At a Dahlem Workshop, scientists are able to pose questions and solicit alternative opinions on contentious issues from colleagues from related fields. The overall goal of a workshop is not necessarily to reach a consensus but rather to identify gaps in knowledge, to find new ways of approaching controversial issues, and to define priorities for future research. This philosophy is implemented at every stage of a workshop: from the selection of the theme to its breakdown in the discussion groups, from the writing of the background papers to the formulation of the group reports.

Workshop topics are proposed by leading scientists and are approved by a scientific board, which is advised by qualified referees. Once a topic has been approved, a Program Advisory Committee of scientists meets approximately one year before the workshop to delineate the scientific parameters of the meeting, select participants, and

---

[1] The Donors' Association for the Promotion of Sciences and Humanities, a foundation created in 1921 in Berlin and supported by German trade and industry to fund basic research in the sciences.
[2] German Science Foundation.

assign them their tasks. Participants are invited on the basis of their scientific standing alone.

Each workshop is organized around four key questions, which are addressed by four discussion groups of approximately ten participants. Lectures or formal presentations are taboo at Dahlem. Instead, concentrated discussion — within a group and between groups — is the means by which maximum communication is achieved. To facilitate this discussion, participants prepare the workshop theme prior to the meeting through the "background papers," the themes and authors of which are chosen by the Program Advisory Committee. These papers specifically review a particular aspect of the group's discussion topic as well as function as a springboard to the group discussion, by introducing controversies or unresolved problem areas.

During the workshop week, each group sets its own agenda to cover the discussion topic. Cross-fertilization between groups is both stressed and encouraged. By the end of the week, in a collective effort, each group has prepared a report reflecting the ideas, opinions, and contentious issues of the group as well as identifying directions for future research and problem areas still in need of resolution.

A Dahlem Workshop initiates and facilitates discussion between a certain number — necessarily restricted — of scientists. Because it is imperative that the discussion and communication should continue after a workshop, we present the results to the scientific community at large in the form of this published volume. In it you will find the revised background papers and group reports, as well as an introduction to the workshop theme itself.

The difference between proceedings of many conventional meetings and this workshop report will be easily discernable. Here, the background papers have not only been reviewed by formal referees, they have been revised according to the many comments and suggestions made by *all* participants. In this sense, they are reviewed more thoroughly than scientific articles in most archival journals. In addition, an extensive editorial procedure ensures a coherent volume. I am sure that you, too, will appreciate the tireless efforts of the many reviewers, authors, and editors.

On their behalf, I sincerely hope that the spirit of this workshop as well as the ideas and controversies raised will stimulate you in your work and future endeavors.

Prof. Dr. Klaus Roth, Director
Dahlem Konferenzen der Freien Universität Berlin
Thielallee 66, D–14195 Berlin, Germany

List of Participants with Fields of Research

ARNAB K. ACHARYA   Harvard Center for Population and Development Studies, 9 Bow Street, Cambridge, MA 02138, U.S.A.

Cost-effectiveness analysis; determinants of burden of disease; inequality of health status

ISAO ARITA   Agency for Cooperation in International Health (ACIH), 4–11–1 Higashi-machi, Kumaoto City 862, Japan

Epidemiology of infectious diseases; management of program for eradicating selective diseases

R. BRUCE AYLWARD   Expanded Programme on Immunization, World Health Organization, 20 Avenue Appia, CH–1211 Geneva 27, Switzerland

Control/eradication of vaccine-preventable diseases, particularly polio, measles, and neonatal tetanus in developing countries; evaluating and reducing the risk of unsafe immunization injections

STEPHEN L. COCHI   Centers for Disease Control and Prevention, National Immunization Program, Mailstop E–05, 1600 Clifton Road, N.E., Atlanta, GA 30333, U.S.A.

Preventive medicine; polio eradication and vaccine — preventable diseases: control and prevention; infectious diseases epidemiology

CIRO A. DE QUADROS   Pan American Health Organization, 525 23rd Street N.W., Washington, D.C. 20037, U.S.A.

Vaccine development and utilization; vaccine-preventable diseases control; public health policy and management

SIEGHART DITTMANN   World Health Organization, Regional Office for Europe, 8 Scherfigsvej, DK–2100 Copenhagen, Denmark

Communicable diseases and immunization programs

WALTER R. DOWDLE   Task Force for Child Survival and Development, One Copenhill, Atlanta, GA 30307, U.S.A.

Infectious diseases; polio eradication

SERGEI G. DROZDOV   Director, Institute of Poliomyelitis, P.O. Institute of Poliomyelitis, 142782 Moscow Region, Russian Federation

Viral diseases (virology and epidemiology); poliomyelitis (prevention, eradication); tick-borne encephalitis, viral gastroenteritis, hemorrhagic fever with renal syndrome

FRANK FENNER   The John Curtin School of Medical Research, The Australian National University, G.P.O. Box 334, Canberra, A.C.T. 2601, Australia

Medical virology; history of biology

STAN O. FOSTER   Division of International Health, Rollins School of Public Health, Rm. 712, 1518 Clifton Road, N.E., Atlanta, GA 30322, U.S.A.

International public health; immunization — policy, training, logistics, evaluation; public health policy, management

JAIME Z. GALVEZ TAN   United Nations Children's Fund, 1086 Del Monte Avenue, Quezon City 1105, Philippines

Community participation in health; health policy development; health human resource development; traditional medicine

PHILIPPE GAXOTTE   MSD Interpharma, 106, Avenue Jean Moulin, F–78170 La Celle Saint Cloud, France

Mectizan® donation program for onchocerciasis control

RICHARD A. GOODMAN   Epidemiology Program Office, MS–C08, Centers for Disease Control and Prevention, 1600 Clifton Road, Atlanta, GA 30333, U.S.A.

Infectious and noninfectious diseases epidemiology; communicating findings of epidemiological research into public health practice; editing internationally circulated public health bulletin

FRANCIS CHAPMAN GRANT   c/o Global 2000, Kotoka International Airport, Private Mailbag, Accra, Ghana

Eradication and control of communicable diseases

MARLENE GYLDMARK   Danish Institute for Health Service, Research and Development, Box 2595, Dampfaergevej 22, DK–2100 Copenhagen Ø, Denmark

Economic evaluation; willingness-to-pay measures; national drug policies

KARL-OTTO HABERMEHL Institut für Klinische und Experimentelle Virologie, Universitätsklinikum Benjamin Franklin, Freie Universität Berlin, Hindenburgdamm 27, D–12203 Berlin, Germany

Clinical virology

ANDREW J. HALL Department of Infectious and Tropical Diseases, London School of Hygiene and Tropical Medicine, Keppel Street, London WC1E 7HT, U.K.

Hepatitis B epidemiology and control; pneumococcal disease epidemiology and control

ROBERT G. HALL Communicable Disease Control Branch, South Australian Health Commission, P.O. Box 6, Rundle Mall, S.A. 5000, Australia

Communicable disease control; mathematical modeling of immunization

ALAN R. HINMAN Task Force for Child Survival and Development, One Copenhill, Atlanta, Georgia 30307, U.S.A.

Infant, child, and adult immunization; economic analysis of preventive measures

DONALD R. HOPKINS Associate Executive Director for Control and Eradication of Disease, The Carter Center/Global 2000, One Copenhill, Atlanta, GA 30307, U.S.A.

Eradication of dracunculiasis; eradication and control of infectious diseases in general

T. JACOB JOHN Department of Clinical Virology, Christian Medical College Hospital, Vellore, Tamil Nadu 632004, India

Epidemiologies of infectious diseases

AEHYUNG KIM World Bank, Room J–9033, 1818 H Street, NW, Washington, D.C. 20433, U.S.A.

Economic impact of non-ocular onchocerciasis: A case study of the Teppi coffee plantation in Ethiopia

MEINRAD A. KOCH Sportforum Straße 11, D–14035 Berlin, Germany

Control of communicable diseases

GRAHAM F. MEDLEY Department of Biological Sciences, University of Warwick, Coventry CV4 7AL, U.K.

Use of mathematical models to design control programs for infectious disease: hepatitis B virus; helminth infection (human and veterinary); nosocomial infections

BJØRN MELGAARD   Global Programmes for Vaccines and Immunization, World Health Organization, CH–1211 Geneva 27, Switzerland

EPI, vaccines, immunization

ALEX S. MULLER   Zandpad 42, NL–3621 NE Breukelen, Netherlands

Epidemiology of infectious diseases

JEAN MICHEL NDIAYE   Regional Adviser/Health (UNICEF), Immeuble Alliance II, 04 B.P. 443 Abidjan, Cote d'Ivoire

Guinea worm eradication; EPI diseases control; health services management

JEAN-MARC OLIVÉ   Expanded Programme on Immunization, World Health Organization, CH–1211 Geneva 27, Switzerland

Control/eradication of vaccine-preventable diseases

VINCENT ORINDA   UNICEF, 3 United Nations Plaza, New York, NY 10017, U.S.A.

ORS (oral rehydration salts) use in diarrhoea

STEPHEN M. OSTROFF   National Center for Infectious Diseases, Mail Stop C12, Rm. 1–6013, Centers for Disease Control and Prevention, 1600 Clifton Road, Atlanta, GA 30333, U.S.A.

Infectious disease epidemiology, control, and prevention

ERIC A. OTTESEN   Filariasis Control (CTD/FIL), Division of Control of Tropical Diseases, World Health Organization, 20, Avenue Appia, CH–1211 Geneva 27, Switzerland

Filariasis/onchocerciasis: control, immunity, pathogenesis

HERBERT A. PIGMAN   Chairman, Task Force on International Advocacy, The Rotary Foundation of Rotary International, 5303 W 850 N, Ambia, IN 47917, U.S.A.

Advocacy for polio eradication

BERNHARD SCHWARTLÄNDER   UNAIDS, 20, Ave. Appia, CH–1211 Geneva 27, Switzerland

Epidemiology and prevention of HIV/AIDS and sexually transmitted diseases

CARL E. TAYLOR   Dept. of International Health, School of Hygiene and Public Health, Johns Hopkins University, 615 N. Wolfe St., Baltimore, MD 21205, U.S.A.

Primary health care

RONALD J. WALDMAN BASICS, Suite 300, 1600 Wilson Blvd., Arlington, VA 22209, U.S.A.

Child health in developing countries

WANG KE-AN Chinese Academy of Preventive Medicine, 27 Nan Wei Road, Beijing 100050, China

Disease prevention and control, especially vaccine-preventable diseases; epidemiology; public health management

HEINZ ZEICHHARDT Institut für Klinische und Experimentelle Virologie, Universitätsklinikum Benjamin Franklin, Freie Universität Berlin, Hindenburgdamm 27, D–12203 Berlin, Germany

Clinical virology; picorna virology

1

Introduction

W.R. DOWDLE[1] and D.R. HOPKINS[2]

[1]Task Force for Child Survival and Development, One Copenhill, Atlanta, GA 30307, U.S.A.
[2]Associate Executive Director for Control and Eradication of Disease,
The Carter Center/Global 2000, One Copenhill, Atlanta, GA 30307, U.S.A.

It is fitting that this Dahlem Workshop was held in 1997, marking the 20th anniversary of the end of smallpox, the first disease of humans to be eradicated. Other seminal related events in the interim include steady progress toward eradication of dracunculiasis and poliomyelitis as well as the work of the International Task Force for Disease Eradication, which evaluated over 80 potential candidate diseases and concluded, in 1993, that six were eradicable. In 1997, the World Health Assembly passed a resolution calling for the "elimination of lymphatic filariasis as a public health problem," and the region of the Americas appears to have almost eliminated indigenous measles. Workshop participants noted the increasing global interest in eradication as evidence of the increasing need to consider the *science* of eradication and its proper role in relation to primary health care development. We believe that the workshop and this volume reflect significant progress toward that end.

The unique format of the Dahlem Workshops provided an ideal setting in which thirty-seven international scientists participated in an interdisciplinary exchange of ideas on aspects of disease eradication for a week in Berlin in March, 1997. It was an extraordinary experience, for which we thank Dr. Klaus Roth and his staff at the Free University of Berlin as well as all of our co-participants.

During the workshop, the group reviewed the history of past and current eradication campaigns, established common definitions (distinguishing among eradication, elimination, and control programs and extinction of an etiologic agent), considered biological and sociopolitical criteria for eradication, the costs and benefits of eradication campaigns, opportunities for strengthening primary health care in the course of eradication efforts, and other aspects of planning and implementing eradication programs. The need for common definitions was vividly illustrated on the eve of the workshop by a WHO press release (March 14, 1997), which asserted that lymphatic filariasis, leprosy, river blindness (onchocerciasis), and Chagas' disease (American trypanosomiasis) could "be eliminated as public health problems within ten years."

The Eradication of Infectious Diseases
Edited by W.R. Dowdle and D.R. Hopkins © 1998 John Wiley & Sons Ltd.

A major goal of this workshop was to find new ways of approaching controversial issues, especially the differing views as to the relative benefits of eradication programs and primary health care programs, and how they are pursued. The authors of background papers were asked to make their manuscripts provocative, in order to stimulate discussion of contentious topics. Authors then revised their papers based on comments received during the workshop. Discussions during the workshop also led us to the unusual but not unprecedented step of commissioning a background paper during the workshop on designing eradication programs to strengthen primary health care. That paper was also subjected to peer review and was revised in light of subsequent written comments by participants.

We believe that eradication programs and primary health care programs are useful means of improving public health, and that the unique contributions of each can and should be complementary. Eradication programs are more easily and efficiently pursued where primary health services are well developed, and should be planned in such a way as to make use of such services where they exist, and to help facilitate their development where they do not yet exist or are weak. Primary health care programs could benefit greatly by including specific disease reduction outcomes among their targets.

The next few decades will surely be exciting ones for disease eradication, beginning with the much larger conference on "Global Disease Elimination and Eradication as Public Health Strategies," which will be held in Atlanta in 1998. We believe and hope this volume will help inform subsequent considerations of these issues and, in doing so, improve the health of all human beings for generations to come.

2

What Is Eradication?

F. FENNER[1], A.J. HALL[2], and W.R. DOWDLE[3]

[1]John Curtin School of Medical Research, Australian National University,
Mills Road, Acton, ACT 200, Australia
[2]London School of Tropical Medicine and Hygiene, Keppel Street,
London WC1E 7HT, U.K.
[3]The Task Force for Child Survival and Development, One Copenhill,
Atlanta, GA 30307, U.S.A.

ABSTRACT

The term *disease eradication* has been commonly used in public health, often inconsistently. This chapter describes the evolution of the term and the need for its appropriate use.

Historically, the first attempts at disease eradication were made with diseases of livestock, always at a country-wide level. The first attempts to eradicate the human diseases hookworm and yellow fever were frustrated by ignorance of the biology of the parasites. Attempts at yellow fever eradication were followed by initially successful campaigns to eradicate the vectors of yellow fever and malaria from particular areas, which with the advent of DDT led to the unsuccessful malaria eradication campaign. The first successful eradication campaign, smallpox, was certified in 1980 and led to proposals for similar global campaigns for poliomyelitis and dracunculiasis. All campaigns need to recognize the need for continuing scientific research to cope with unexpected problems. Some authors have contended that if a disease is eradicated, another will arise to fill that ecologic niche. We believe that there is no basis for this belief.

The task before this workshop was to consider the historical use of the term *eradication*, as well as the associated terms of *control*, *elimination*, and *extinction* and to develop appropriate definitions to facilitate communication and promote meaningful discussions of the issues.

INTRODUCTION

Almost 200 years ago, Jenner (1801) published a short pamphlet in which he made the statement: ". . . it now becomes too manifest to admit of controversy, that the annihilation of the Small Pox, the most dreadful scourge of the human species, must be the result of this practice." If we equate "annihilation" with "eradication," Jenner was the first proponent of the notion that it would prove possible to eradicate (literally, "to tear out by the roots") an infectious disease. Pasteur was probably the first to use

The Eradication of Infectious Diseases
Edited by W.R. Dowdle and D.R. Hopkins © 1998 John Wiley & Sons Ltd.

the term eradication when he wrote, "It is within the power of man to eradicate infection from the earth" (Dubos and Dubos 1953). Gradually the term "eradication" came into wider use and was given a variety of definitions, applying to diseases of livestock as well as to diseases of humans.

ERADICATION AS APPLIED TO DISEASES OF LIVESTOCK

The first serious efforts to get rid of infectious diseases were focused on diseases of livestock, and their spatial dimension was that of one of the wealthy developed countries. The desired result was called "eradication," conceived on a national, not a global, scale. Indeed, although country-wide eradication is the proclaimed aim of most developed countries when faced with exotic diseases of livestock, no proposal has ever been made for the global eradication of any such disease.

Bovine Pleuropneumonia

Bovine pleuropneumonia, caused by *Mycoplasma mycoides*, had been known in Asia and Africa for hundreds of years before it became widespread in Europe during the early part of the 19th century. In the mid-1850s it was spread to the United States and Australia in cattle imported from Europe. Initially restricted to the eastern states of the U.S., by 1886 it had reached Illinois, Kentucky, and Missouri. The need to control this disease led to the establishment of the Bureau of Animal Industry of the U.S. Department of Agriculture in 1884. In 1887, Congress made funds available to the Bureau to eradicate the disease, and by September, 1892, the U.S. was free of the disease.

Introduced into the southern state of Victoria, Australia, in 1858, bovine pleuropneumonia had spread into New South Wales, Queensland, and the Northern Territory by 1880, and into Western Australia in 1897. Control by vaccination was begun in 1862, but a high-quality vaccine was not available until 1937. The disease was readily eradicated from the concentrated herds of southern Australia, but control presented great difficulties in the vast cattle runs of the North. However, the combination of widespread vaccination with an effective vaccine, the control of movement of cattle, and the declaration of "free areas" led to its elimination from the whole country in 1968 (Pierce 1969).

Other Animal Diseases

Several other diseases of domestic animals, including foot-and-mouth disease, rinderpest, and Newcastle disease of chickens, have occurred for centuries in Africa and/or Asia and have periodically spread to Europe, North America, and Australia. These incursions have usually been quickly recognized and the disease eradicated from the affected countries, usually by widespread vaccination, slaughter of diseased and exposed animals, or a combination. This procedure can sometimes be very expensive, e.g., with foot-and-mouth disease; however, the loss of markets caused by the presence of this disease can be vastly more costly.

ERADICATION AS APPLIED TO DISEASES OF HUMANS

For technical and administrative reasons, achieving Jenner's goal of smallpox eradication required 176 years. This is not the place to discuss the technical reasons, but it is important to draw attention to an important administrative reason, namely the requirement that information on the incidence of human infectious diseases should be "globalized." Although this began in a rudimentary way with the establishment of the Health Commission of the League of Nations after the First World War, it was not until the World Health Organization (WHO) was established in 1948 that it was possible to obtain information on disease incidence in every country of the world. Even then, this information was often woefully incomplete, but at least a mechanism was in place to provide figures against which progress toward global eradication could be measured. However, long before this, the lack of information did not prevent some enthusiasts from promoting the concept of eradication of several different diseases.

The first disease to be considered seriously for global eradication was hookworm. An eradication program was mounted in 1909 and followed soon afterwards by a program for global eradication of yellow fever. As we now know, neither was a reasonable candidate, but at the time the programs were initiated, inadequate scientific knowledge, coupled with a visionary outlook and excessive optimism, made them appear suitable. As the programs progressed, it became increasingly evident that disease eradication was a formidable task and for many diseases, an unattainable goal.

Hookworm

Early this century Dr. C.W. Stiles, an official in the U.S. Health Service, conceived the idea of interrupting the spread of hookworm in the southern states of the U.S. by a systematic campaign in which infected persons would be identified by stool examinations and their infections cured by drug therapy. At the same time, the construction of sanitary privies would prevent fecal contamination of the soil and thus break the transmission cycle, in which the larvae enter the body through the skin of the feet, migrate to the intestinal mucosae where they feed on blood in the capillaries, and shed eggs that are passed in the feces to the soil, where they develop into larvae. This plan appealed to the advisers of John D. Rockefeller, and the Rockefeller Sanitary Commission for the Eradication of Hookworm was established in 1909, with Stiles as director (Grove 1990).

By 1914 the Commission had screened more than 2 million persons, of whom 500,000 were treated in mobile dispensaries, and more than 250,000 rural homes had been inspected by sanitary personnel. In 1913 the Rockefeller Foundation was established, with an International Health Commission into which the Rockefeller Sanitary Commission was incorporated. As its first initiative, the Foundation decided "to extend to other countries and people the work of eradicating hookworm disease as opportunity offers, and so far as practicable to follow up . . . with the establishment of public sanitation." In the following years cooperative programs extended to 52 countries on 6 continents and to 29 island groups.

However, although the improvement of health in areas that had been treated was obvious, no field studies had been conducted to determine whether hookworm had actually been eradicated. When such studies were eventually conducted, they showed that the infection rates had not significantly diminished, although those infected had fewer worms and thus less illness due to the disease. It was clear that the biology of the hookworm was far more complex than had been anticipated.

Yellow Fever

Recurrent severe epidemics of yellow fever had plagued cities of the southern United States since the 17th century, but it never became endemic there. By the end of the 19th century it was believed that most of these epidemics were the consequence of importations from Cuba, hence when Cuba was occupied by United States forces in 1898, yellow fever control was of special interest to the health authorities. The Yellow Fever Commission, set up in 1900 and directed by Major Walter Reed, very quickly made a number of brilliant discoveries, notably that it was transmitted by the urban mosquito, *Aedes aegypti,* thus opening the way for control of yellow fever (Reed 1902).

The Chief Sanitary Officer for Cuba, Major W.C. Gorgas, established a comprehensive scheme to screen patients and destroy breeding places of *Aedes aegypti,* and the last case of yellow fever occurred in Havana in September 1901, only 8 months after the campaign had begun. Heartened by this result, Gorgas (1911) reported to General Leonard Wood that: "I look forward in the future to a time when yellow fever will have entirely disappeared as a disease to which man is subject . . . ." This attitude was strengthened by the elimination of yellow fever from Panama and then from Rio de Janeiro. A few years later, after a visit to Asia, where the vector was widespread but the disease did not occur, the Director of the International Health Commission of the Rockefeller Foundation became interested in extending measures against yellow fever on a worldwide scale. Delayed by the First World War, *Aedes aegypti* eradication programs were launched by the Foundation in 1918 in many countries in Central and South America, and for almost a year, from April, 1927, to March, 1928, no cases of yellow fever were reported from anywhere in the Americas. The Rockefeller Foundation prepared for programs in Africa, establishing laboratories to study the disease in West Africa and later in Uganda.

The seemingly unbroken triumph in South America was interrupted later in 1928 by outbreaks in northeast Brazil, in Rio de Janeiro, and then in Colombia and Venezuela. These dramatized the need for more effective disease surveillance but presaged a more serious discovery, namely that there was a jungle reservoir of the disease, transmitted not by *Aedes aegypti* but by mosquitoes that ordinarily lived in the forest canopy. This underlined one of the most important principles in the selection of human diseases as candidates for global eradication — this was impossible if there was an animal reservoir (Warren 1951).

Aedes aegypti

The director of the Rockefeller Foundation *Aedes aegypti* control campaign in Brazil in the 1930s was Dr. F.L. Soper, an ardent and forceful proponent of disease eradication. With the discovery of jungle yellow fever, it was clear that global eradication of yellow fever could not be achieved, but Soper saw that human cases could be greatly reduced if *Aedes aegypti*, the vector of urban yellow fever, was eliminated. Eradication of the mosquito was a much more difficult proposition than reduction to a level that could not sustain continuous transmission of yellow fever, but Soper had in place a highly disciplined and well-organized program, and in 1934 he proposed that the Foundation should support such an objective. A Cooperative Yellow Fever Service was established by the Foundation and the Brazilian government, but after some delay the Foundation felt that it called for too great a commitment, and in 1939 it withdrew its support. However, by that time the Cooperative Service had eliminated the mosquito from several states and many cities, and in 1942 the Brazilian government's National Yellow Fever Service assumed responsibility for "the complete eradication of the species." By 1961 Soper (1963) was able to report that *Aedes aegypti* had been almost completely eradicated from the Americas, "the principal delinquent in this international effort being the United States of America." However, it was not to last, and beginning in the late 1970s many areas were reinfested. By the late 1980s *Aedes aegypti* was reestablished in many cities in South and Central America, as demonstrated by a succession of epidemics of dengue involving multiple serotypes and the occurrence of hemorrhagic dengue (Monath and Heinz 1996).

Anopheles gambiae

Anopheles gambiae, an African mosquito, is an exceptionally efficient vector of malaria. Soon after the establishment in 1930 of a rapid mail service between Dakar, in Senegal, and Natal, in northeast Brazil, epidemic malaria occurred in an area of a few square kilometers in which the mosquito was first found. It was readily controlled in Natal, but in 1938 severe epidemics occurred over an area of some 31,000 square kilometers. Soper proposed that the Rockefeller Foundation and the Brazilian government should cooperate in a program to eradicate *Anopheles gambiae* from Brazil. Rather reluctantly, the Foundation agreed, and Soper was placed in control (Soper and Wilson 1943). With a staff of about 4,000, the boundaries of the area were determined and all vehicles entering or leaving the area were fumigated. In the infested area, Paris green was used for larval control and pyrethrum for spraying houses. These measures reduced but did not eliminate the vector population during the wet season, but when the dry season came control was converted to eradication, the last *Anopheles gambiae* being discovered less than two years after the program was launched.

In 1944, showing that this was no fluke, Soper took charge of a campaign to eradicate *Anopheles gambiae* from Egypt, into which it had been introduced in 1942. Using the same procedures as in Brazil, he was again successful, the last focus being eliminated in February, 1945. These successes reinforced Soper's conviction that selective species eradication was often a sound and less expensive approach than control of the vector and the disease. With his election in 1947 as Director of the Pan American Sanitary Bureau (later the Pan American Health Organization), Soper had the opportunity to put his ideas into practice, and he was an enthusiastic proponent of eradication of *Aedes aegypti* from the Americas, and subsequently of campaigns to eradicate malaria, yaws, and smallpox from the Americas, and later, through WHO, globally.

Malaria

In spite of having dismissed a proposal for the global eradication of smallpox, made by the then Director-General of WHO, Dr. Brock Chisholm in 1953, the World Health Assembly approved the vastly more difficult project of malaria eradication in 1955. As discussed in a recent conference (Bynum and Fantini 1997), this proposal was driven by the spectacular success of DDT for mosquito control and the fact that by 1951 scattered reports were coming in about mosquito resistance to DDT. It was felt to be essential to capitalize on the use of DDT before its effectiveness was eroded by developing resistance. Although a number of successes were recorded, in islands, in some Mediterranean countries, and in the Americas, the campaign was a failure, in spite of the expenditure of some US$ 2 billion by WHO and other international agencies. As some said, by concentrating on DDT and neglecting other methods of malaria control, the campaign eliminated malariologists, not malaria. As Jeffery (1976) observed: "The *science* of malaria control, developed slowly and painfully from the beginning of the century to a relatively high state of sophistication, was almost overnight converted to the rather simplistic *technology* of malaria eradication, which basically required that one know how to deliver 2 grams of something to 2 square metres of a sometimes elusive interior wall, and to manage a hopefully ever-diminishing Kardex file of cases."

Yaws

Yaws, caused by the spirochaete *Treponema pertenue,* is transmitted by direct non-sexual contact from person to person, and causes chronic, deforming and incapacitating lesions. In 1949 it was found in Haiti, long a highly endemic area, that yaws, unlike syphilis, could be cured by a single injection of long-acting penicillin. Under Soper's influence, the Pan American Sanitary Bureau passed a resolution committing itself to yaws eradication in the Americas. Individual patients were diagnosed by inspection and given penicillin, or where the disease was widespread, the entire population was treated. The results were immediate and dramatic, but there were occasional latent infections and sometimes such patients relapsed and transmission resumed.

WHO never made a commitment to yaws eradication, although the Expert Committee on Treponematoses strongly supported such an effort. However, between 1948 and 1968 WHO and other international agencies invested more than US$ 9 million in 61 countries and territories to support programs for the control of syphilis and yaws by treatment with penicillin. Programs designed to achieve country-wide elimination of yaws were launched in 49 countries, and although they were remarkably effective, the disease was eliminated in only a few of the smaller countries (Yekutiel 1981). There was far more low-level persistent infection and transmission than had been supposed, and follow-up surveillance was not good enough to find and treat such cases.

Smallpox

Following Brock Chisholm's abortive attempt in 1953, a successful proposal for the global eradication of smallpox, introduced by the Soviet Union, was accepted by the World Health Assembly in 1958. It was based on the concept, successfully demonstrated in many countries of Europe and in the U.S.S.R., that if a level of 80% vaccination could be achieved, herd immunity would ensure that transmission would be interrupted. The main problem, as then envisaged, was to ensure that all endemic countries received adequate supplies of vaccine and used it throughout their populations.

By 1964 it was apparent that this strategy, while successful in many smaller countries, would not succeed in the Indian subcontinent. In 1966 the World Health Assembly therefore provided base funding of US$ 2.4 million annually to support a ten-year intensified smallpox eradication program. D.A. Henderson was appointed to lead the project. The key features of the program that he set up were an intensive system of surveillance and containment in the endemic countries, supervised by international personnel but carried out by the national health services, the provision of adequate supplies of high-quality vaccine, the continuation in endemic countries of routine vaccination designed to achieve at least 80% vaccination levels, and the availability of backup scientific expertise for diagnosis, evaluation of vaccine quality, and the investigation of unexpected difficulties. "Surveillance and containment" were vital to the success of the intensified program. It was a procedure by which efforts were made to ensure that all cases were diagnosed promptly and in which such diagnoses were followed up by discovery of the source of the case and ring vaccination of persons in the immediate environment of both the index case and the case from which the infection had been acquired. The provision of adequate quantities of vaccine was ensured by developing a guidebook for vaccine production, ensuring that vaccine producers in endemic countries used reliable production methods, and encouraging large-scale donations of vaccine from countries able to make them. The provision of high-quality vaccines was somewhat more difficult. Independent laboratories were eventually used to ensure that all vaccines used in the eradication program met WHO standards for potency, heat stability, and freedom from pathogenic bacteria (Fenner et al. 1988).

Helminthic Diseases

Following the success of the smallpox eradication program, a meeting was held in Washington, D.C., to consider other candidates for global eradication (Stuart-Harris et al. 1982). Schistosomiasis was one of the diseases discussed at length (Strickland 1982). However, helminths differ from microparasites in that they do not multiply in their animal host. Most people harboring worms carry only a small load and are perfectly healthy, hence there is a vast undetectable reservoir. Control by treatment of individual sick persons, who have heavy infestations, is almost always the preferred strategy (Warren 1982).

In the discussion that followed Warren's paper, Hopkins (1982) pointed out that Guinea worm disease (dracunculiasis) was an exception, in that one worm produced a serious, readily diagnosable disease. Moreover, the disease was localized to Africa, the Indian subcontinent, and parts of the Middle East, and within these areas it was highly focal in distribution. Since humans are infected by swallowing water containing minute crustaceans (genus *Cyclops*), which can be removed by filtering water through muslin, control was feasible at a relatively low cost. In recognition of these epidemiologic facts, in 1991 the WHO endorsed a plan to eradicate dracunculiasis globally by 1995, proceeding on a country-by-country basis. The strategies were outlined by Hopkins and Ruiz-Tiben (1991). After several years, elimination from several countries was achieved, and the International Commission for the Certification of Dracunculiasis Eradication held its first meeting in March, 1996.

Poliomyelitis and Measles

At the Washington, D.C., meeting measles was regarded as the most likely next candidate, largely because the absence of inapparent infections made surveillance much simpler than in poliomyelitis. However, following the success of the proposal of the Pan American Health Organization in May, 1985, to interrupt the transmission of wild poliovirus in the Americas, in 1988 the World Health Assembly resolved to eradicate poliomyelitis from the world by the year 2000. The target for measles was the more modest one of a 95% reduction in measles deaths and a 90% reduction in measles cases by 1995. The poliomyelitis eradication program is well on track, and the reduction of measles prompted a consultation between the Pan American Health Organization, WHO, and the Centers for Disease Control and Prevention to set a tentative target of 2010 for global measles eradication.

THE DEFINITION OF ERADICATION

The foregoing brief historical review reveals that eradication has had different meanings at different times with different diseases. Eradication has often been used to describe what is now considered control or elimination. Cockburn (1961) proposed eradication to mean the extinction of the disease pathogen. Soper (1962) proposed the objective of eradication to be the complete elimination "of the occurrence of a given disease, even in the absence of all preventive measures." Andrews and Langmuir (1963) used the term to mean control of an infection to the point at which transmission ceased within a specified area.

For diseases of livestock, it is quite efficient for "eradication" to be achieved in a "specified area" as small as a country (especially a country with few international borders), for importations can to a large extent be prevented by quarantine, and accidental introductions can be controlled relatively easily by slaughter of diseased and exposed animals. Neither mechanism is available for diseases of humans. Soper's definition is global. It requires that there is no possibility of reintroducing the pathogen from another geographic area; eradication and its benefits are permanent. For most diseases of humans with a distribution in many different countries, "regional eradication" is an oxymoron because of the ever-present risk of importation of the pathogen and the continuing need for control measures. For such situations it is better to use the term "regional elimination," which is often a necessary preliminary to attempts at global eradication.

Soper's definition also directly addresses the eventual removal of control measures, which is crucial to the resultant economic benefits. Hinman (1984) proposed an important modification of the definition by adding that eradication must be due to deliberate efforts (rather than the disappearance of a disease by chance). Further modifications were made by the International Task Force for Disease Eradication (CDC 1993), which defined eradication as "reduction of the worldwide incidence of a disease to zero as a result of deliberate efforts, obviating the necessity for further control measures."

Extinction of the Disease Pathogen

So far, none of the definitions, except Cockburn's (1961), has addressed the issue of extinction of the pathogen from nature. For some pathogens with complex life cycles, such as Guinea worm *(Dracunculus medinensis)*, eradication is synonymous with extinction, since humans are essential for the life cycle, but the worm cannot replicate in humans. Because most bacterial or viral pathogens can replicate in the laboratory, in media, in cells, or in experimental animals, extinction is far more complex. Extinction requires documented destruction of all known existing stocks and potentially infectious materials.

Extinction was not the intitial objective of the WHO Smallpox Eradication Unit when it was established in 1967. Its goal was the interruption of transmission, which in smallpox could be equated with the total disappearance of the disease. The reason for restricting the goal was that at that time variola virus was used for diagnosis in many laboratories, all over the world, and it was routine practice for virologists to keep reference samples stored in their deep-freeze cabinets. When it came to the certification of eradication, it was thought that it would be impossible to assure the world community that every vial of the virus in deep freeze cabinets in every country in the world had been destroyed. However, WHO made a major effort to reduce progressively the number of laboratories holding the virus, as the need for it disappeared with progressive country-wide eradication. The number of laboratories was reduced from 75 in 1975 to 18 in 1977 (the year of the last case) and then to two: the WHO Collaborating Centers for Smallpox Diagnosis in Atlanta and Moscow (now in Koltsovo).

Extinction has not been easily achieved. In 1986, the WHO Committee on Orthopoxvirus Infections recommended that since by this time cloned fragments of the genome of several strains of variola virus were available, the remaining stocks of virus or scab material should be destroyed (WHO 1986). WHO did not act on this recommendation, but in 1990, when the art of nucleotide sequencing was much more advanced, WHO called the committee together again to discuss a project for sequencing the genome of a few representative strains, as a prelude to destruction in December, 1993 (Mahy et al. 1991; WHO 1992). By that date the complete sequence of two strains of smallpox virus and nonconserved sequences of several other strains had been determined (Massung et al. 1994). However, the committee's recommendation was twice deferred, initially because of objections by some scientists and later for political reasons. The decision to destroy laboratory stocks of smallpox virus was urged by the Committee on Orthopoxvirus Infections because although smallpox virus was not a good agent for biological warfare between traditional armies, it was an excellent terrorist weapon. To answer objections by scientists that the sequencing had revealed a number of interesting questions about pathogenesis, members of the committee pointed out that these could be answered by using another orthopoxvirus such as ectromelia or vaccinia virus in the very convenient host animal, the laboratory mouse (WHO 1994). The prospect of keeping stocks of smallpox virus microbiologically and militarily secure, forever, in an insecure world, did not, in the committee's view, justify the risk (Dowdle 1995). Eventually, in May, 1996, the World Health Assembly agreed that all stocks should be destroyed in June, 1999. It was argued at the Assembly that retention in the Russian Federation and the United States for another three years would provide a counterbalance to terrorism and allow time for more sensitive methods of virus detection to be developed.

As the poliovirus eradication target date approaches, another emotional debate has surfaced in the scientific community on the fate of the laboratory stocks, although no national security measures have yet emerged. The problem that polioviruses might be used as biological weapons does not arise, but laboratory infections are well documented, and virus that might escape from a laboratory would spread explosively in unimmunized populations (Dowdle and Birmingham 1997). Arguments for retention of poliovirus stocks are (a) that the risks to public health are exaggerated, since stocks of vaccine could be stored and made available if necessary, and (b) that poliovirus should be retained for future research benefits and the assurance of biodiversity (although it could be argued that biodiversity requires that to be living, the virus should continue to occupy its natural ecologic niche — which is the human body!).

Nevertheless, a good argument can be made that in principle any virus whose sequence is known could be re-created in the laboratory. Knowing the sequences of related orthopoxviruses, genes that appear to be peculiar to smallpox could be transferred to, for example, vaccinia or monkeypox virus. However, proving the virulence for humans of the newly created virus would be another matter. Poliovirus has a much smaller genome than smallpox virus and has been used for many years as a laboratory model for basic studies in virology. The vast amount of published information, the widespread laboratory experience with poliovirus and the simplicity of its genome make it a prime theoretical candidate for re-creation. Virulence could be demonstrated in monkeys, but transmissibility in humans could only be proved in humans.

Regardless of theoretical feasibility, the re-creation of smallpox virus or poliovirus in the laboratory for malevolent purposes requires vastly more planning, resources, and scientific expertise than taking stocks from a freezer, or reintroducing the disease through a laboratory accident.

The prospect of measles virus being next in line for global eradication raises additional questions. It seems to us that disposition of laboratory stocks should be considered ad hoc as each candidate faces eradication, bearing in mind that early discussions will be needed as to who makes the decision and how it is enforced.

ERADICATION AND THE NEED FOR LABORATORY CONTAINMENT

Because pathogen extinction seems to provoke such strong philosophic arguments, the simplest political response has been to postpone indefinitely the destruction of laboratory stocks. The questions then becomes one of appropriate laboratory containment. For smallpox, the risk of a laboratory-associated outbreak was demonstrated less than a year after the last natural case occurred. In 1978 an outbreak was associated with a laboratory in the United Kingdom and resulted in two cases of smallpox, with one death, and the self-inflicted death of a laboratory investigator (Her Majesty's Stationery Office 1980). In consequence, WHO requested all countries still holding virus to send it to one of the designated WHO Laboratories in the United States (Atlanta) or the then Soviet Union (Moscow). Nevertheless, the risk remains that with storage for an indefinite time even one or other of these laboratories may become targets for terrorist attacks.

The consolidation of poliovirus stocks under appropriate laboratory containment poses a much greater challenge than for smallpox virus, since wild and/or vaccine polioviruses are to be found in public health, clinical, research, and industry laboratories in many countries of the world as known stocks or unidentified clinical specimens. WHO has under consideration a proposal to convene technical advisory groups in 1997 to draft interim post-eradication containment and surveillance guidelines. The difficulty of requiring reliable evidence of the absence of poliovirus from all but a small number of designated laboratories is a strong reason for having a definition for the global eradication of poliomyelitis which does not require the demonstration of extinction of the pathogen.

IF A PATHOGEN IS ERADICATED, WILL ANOTHER FILL THAT ECOLOGIC NICHE?

Some have argued that it is pointless to attempt to eradicate a pathogen because the "ecologic niche" thus created will be filled by an etiologic agent of equal or greater pathogenicity. There was natural concern when monkeypox virus was recognized as causing disease in humans in Africa in 1970. Subsequent genetic studies have shown that it was a very rare disease and that most cases were probably derived from squirrels or monkeys, the secondary attack rate among unvaccinated contacts being 7.47% (Jezek and Fenner 1988). Epidemiologic analysis clearly demonstrated that the transmissibility of monkeypox precluded establishment of the infection in human populations except as a sporadic zoonosis (Fine et al. 1988). Restriction mapping and sequence comparisons of a conserved region of the genomes of both viruses provide strong evidence that monkeypox virus is not ancestral to smallpox virus (Douglass and Dumbell 1992). Monkeypox cases continue to occur, especially in Zaire, where there was a relatively large outbreak (about 100 cases) in the Sankuru region of eastern Zaire in 1996, two-thirds of which may have been acquired from other infected persons (WHO 1996).

Speculation about possible replacement pathogens for the polioviruses has involved the cell receptors for these viruses found in humans, which appear to be used almost exclusively by polioviruses (Wimmer et al. 1996). There are no known biologic principles that might drive the evolution of other viruses to use these receptors.

Further reasons to be skeptical about the "ecologic niche" hypothesis are provided by the history of the freedom from smallpox of several countries (e.g., Australia) for as long as 80 years, the absence of diseases like foot-and-mouth disease, rinderpest, hog cholera, and other diseases of domestic animals in many countries where they have occurred, but have been eliminated, and the absence of a "replacement" of wild polioviruses from several countries from which they were eliminated many years ago.

There is no doubt that "new" infections of humans will continue to emerge, as with increasing population pressure human beings come into closer contact with animals or an environment that carry previously unknown viruses, bacteria, or parasites that can infect humans (Lederberg et al. 1992; Morse 1993). However, with known human pathogens, the basic question is one of weighing the benefits of eradicating it versus the hypothetical risks of a "replacement," by which is meant by those who argue the case for the filling of a vacated ecologic niche, a pathogen that has the same ecologic characteristics as the agent that has been eradicated.

THE NEED FOR A RESEARCH CAPACITY

Perhaps the most important lessons from past eradication programs has been recognition that problems that can only be resolved by research will arise in all eradication programs, especially with diseases as complex as malaria. This point was fully appreciated by Henderson when the intensified smallpox eradication program was undertaken in 1967, and he insisted from the outset that he could call on expertise in the virology of the poxviruses. It was only such expertise that could dispose of the reports on "whitepox," (variola virus supposed to have been isolated from wild animals in Africa), and research conducted in parallel with the program resulted in the recognition of a new disease, human monkeypox, the development of a new method of vaccination, the bifurcated needle, and the assurance of high-quality vaccine.

Because the scientific challenges were greater, research has been even more important in the Poliomyelitis Eradication Program. Methods were needed, and found, for quickly distinguishing wild from vaccine strains of poliovirus (Kew et al. 1990), and highly sensitive methods were developed for characterizing viruses isolated from stool specimens. Unanticipated research questions continue to arise. With the growing confidence that wild poliovirus can be eradicated, research is currently being directed toward developing an appropriate strategy for stopping polio immunization. Questions that remain to be answered include those related to persistent shedding of vaccine-derived virus among some immunocompromised vacinees and the possible circulation of revertant vaccine-derived viruses in the population. With any eradication program, progress brings new questions and new research challenges.

REFERENCES

Andrews, J.M., and A.D. Langmuir. 1963. The philosophy of disease eradication. *Am. J. Pub. Hlth.* **53**:1–6.

Bynum, W.L., and B. Fantini, eds. 1997. Strategies against malaria: Eradication or control? *Parasitologia*, in press.

CDC (Centers for Disease Control and Prevention). 1993. Recommendations of the International Task Force for Disease Eradication. *Morbid. Mortal. Wkly. Rep.* **42 (RR–16)**:1–38.

Cockburn, T.A. 1961. Eradication of infectious diseases. *Science* **133**:1050–1058.

Douglass, N., and K. Dumbell. 1992. Independent evolution of monkeypox and variola viruses. *J. Virol.* **66**:7565–7567.

Dowdle, W.R. 1995. Destruction of the smallpox virus: Why the debate? *Clin. Microbiol. Newsl.* **17**:101–102.

Dowdle, W.R., and M. Birmingham. 1997. The biologic principles of poliovirus eradication. *J. Infec. Dis.* **175**:286–292.

Dubos, R., and J. Dubos. 1953. The White Plague: Tuberculosis, Man and Society. London: Gollancz.

Fenner, F., D.A. Henderson, I. Arita, Z. Jezek, and I.D. Ladnyi. 1988. Smallpox and Its Eradication. Geneva: WHO.

Fine, P.E.M., Z. Jezek, B. Grab, and H. Dixon. 1988. The transmission potential of monkeypox in human populations. *Intl. J. Epidemiol.* **17**:643–650.

Gorgas, W.C. 1911. Report of Major W.C. Gorgas, Medical Corps, United States Army — July 12, 1902. U.S. Senate Document No. 822, pp. 234–238. Washington, D.C.: GPO. Quoted in Fenner et al. (1988).

Grove, D.I. 1990. A History of Human Helminthology, pp. 528–531. Wallingford, U.K.: CAB International.

Her Majesty's Stationery Office. 1980. Report on an Investigation into the Cause of the 1978 Birmingham Smallpox Occurrence. London: Her Majesty's Stationery Office.

Hinman, A.R. 1984. Prospects for disease eradication or elimination. *NY St. J. Med.* **84**:502–506.

Hopkins, D.R. 1982. Comment after G.T. Strickland. *Rev. Infec. Dis.* **4**:960–961.

Hopkins, D.R., and E. Ruiz-Tiben. 1991. Strategies for dracunculiasis eradication. *Bull. WHO* **69**:533–540.

Jeffrey, G.M. 1976. Malaria control in the twentieth century. *Am. J. Trop. Med. Hyg.* **25**:361–371.

Jenner, E. 1801. The Origin of Vaccine Inoculation. London: Shury.

Jezek, Z., and F. Fenner. 1988. Human monkeypox. *Monogr. Virol.* **17**.

Kew, O.M., B.K. Nottay, R. Rico-Hesse, and M.A. Pallansch. 1990. Molecular epidemiology of wild poliovirus transmission. *Appl. Virol. Res.* **2**:199–221.

Lederberg, J., R.E. Shope, and S.C. Oaks, eds. 1992. Emerging Infections. Washington, D.C.: National Academy Press.

Mahy, B.W.J., J.J. Esposito, and J.C. Venter. 1991. Sequencing the smallpox virus genome. Prelude to the destruction of a virus species. *ASM News* **57**:1225–1226.

Massung, R.F., L. Liu, and J. Qi, et al. 1994. The complete genome of smallpox variola major virus strain Bangladesh. *Virology* **201**:215–240.

Monath, T.P., and F.X. Heinz. 1996. Flaviviruses. In: Fields Virology, ed. B.N. Fields, D.M. Knipe, and P.M. Howley, p. 1021. Philadelphia: Lippincott-Raven.

Morse, S.S., ed. 1993. Emerging Viruses. New York: Oxford Univ. Press.

Pierce, A.E. 1969. Progress in the campaign to eradicate bovine contagious pleuropneumonia from Australia. *Bull. Off. Intl. Epiz.* **71**:1313–1328.

Reed, W. 1902. Recent researches concerning the etiology, propagation, and prevention of yellow fever, by the United States Army Commission. *J. Hyg.* **2**:101–119.

Soper, F.L. 1962. Problems to be solved if the eradication of tuberculosis is to be realized. *Am. J. Publ. Hlth.* **52**:734–745.

Soper, F.L. 1963. The elimination of urban yellow fever in the Americas through the eradication of *Aedes aegypti*. *Am. J. Publ. Hlth.* **53**:6–26.

Soper, F.L., and D.B. Wilson. 1943. *Anopheles gambiae* in Brazil 1930–1940. New York: Rockefeller Foundation.

Strickland, G.T. 1982. Schistosomiasis: Eradication or control? *Rev. Infec. Dis.* **4**:951–954.

Stuart-Harris, C., K.A. Western, and E.C. Chamberlayne. 1982. Can infectious diseases be eradicated? *Rev. Infec. Dis.* **4**:913–984.

Warren, A.J. 1951. Landmarks in the conquest of yellow fever. In: Yellow Fever, ed. G.K. Strode, pp. 1–37. New York: McGraw-Hill.

Warren, K.S. 1982. The present impossibility of eradicating the omnipresent worm. *Rev. Infec. Dis.* **4**:955–959.

WHO (World Health Organization). 1986. Committee on Orthopoxvirus Infections. Report of fourth meeting. *Wkly. Epidemiol. Rec.* **1**:289–293.

WHO. 1992. Post-smallpox eradication policies. *Wkly. Epidemiol. Rec.* **1**:3–4.

WHO. 1994. Report of the meeting of the ad hoc Committee on Orthopoxvirus Infections. Programme on Viral, Bacterial Diseases and Immunology. CDS/BVI/94.3.

WHO. 1996. Monkeypox. Zaire. *Wkly. Epidemiol. Rec.* **43**:326.

Wimmer, E., J. Harber, and G. Bernhardt, et al. 1996. Genetic variation and identity of picornaviruses: What is the probability of the emergence of poliovirus type 4? *Abstr. Xth Intl. Congr. Virology,* Jerusalem.

Yekutiel, P. 1981. Lessons from the big eradication campaigns. *World Hlth. For.* **2**:465–481.

3

Lessons from Previous Eradication Programs

A.R. HINMAN[1] and D.R. HOPKINS[2]

[1]Senior Consultant for Public Health Programs, The Task Force for Child Survival and Development, One Copenhill, Atlanta, Georgia 30307, U.S.A.
[2]Associate Executive Director for Control and Eradication of Disease, The Carter Center/Global 2000, One Copenhill, Atlanta, GA 30307, U.S.A.

ABSTRACT

We have reviewed personal and published experiences with one successful eradication program (smallpox), two apparently successful eradication programs which are still underway (dracunculiasis and poliomyelitis), and three unsuccessful programs (malaria, yaws, and yellow fever/*Aedes aegypti*). We have also drawn on the work of the International Task Force for Disease Eradication. We draw ten main lessons from these experiences:

- Understand the natural history of the disease thoroughly.
- Consult widely before embarking on eradication.
- Initiate surveillance early and use surveillance information to guide program strategy.
- Eradication programs require a vertical approach.
- Remain open minded and flexible; expect the unexpected.
- Some countries will need more help than others.
- Coordination of external donors is essential.
- Political commitments from all levels are essential.
- Inspire enthusiasm, but don't declare success prematurely.
- Set a specific target date for eradication.

A final lesson is that eradication of some diseases is possible, but it is not easy. Eradication is the ultimate in communicable disease control and in sustainability.

INTRODUCTION

In preparing this report, we have reviewed personal and published experiences with one successful eradication program (smallpox), two apparently successful eradication programs which are still underway (dracunculiasis and poliomyelitis), and three unsuccessful programs (malaria, yaws, and yellow fever/*Aedes aegypti*). We have also

The Eradication of Infectious Diseases
Edited by W.R. Dowdle and D.R. Hopkins © 1998 John Wiley & Sons Ltd.

Table 3.1 Criteria for assessing eradicability of diseases and conditions.

Scientific Feasibility

- Epidemiologic vulnerability (e.g., existence of nonhuman reservoir; ease of spread; natural cyclical decline in prevalence; naturally induced immunity; ease of diagnosis; and duration of any relapse potential).
- Effective, practical intervention available (e.g., vaccine or other primary preventive, curative treatment, and means of eliminating vector). Ideally, intervention should be effective, safe, inexpensive, long-lasting, and easily deployed.
- Demonstrated feasibility of elimination (e.g., documented elimination from island or other geographic unit).

Political Will/Popular Support

- Perceived burden of the disease (e.g., extent, deaths, other effects; true burden may not be perceived; the reverse of benefits expected to accrue from eradication; relevance to rich and poor countries).
- Expected cost of eradication (especially in relation to perceived burden from the disease).
- Synergy of eradication efforts with other interventions (e.g., potential for added benefits or savings or spin-off effects).
- Necessity for eradication rather than control.

Source: ITFDE (CDC 1993)

drawn on the work of the International Task Force for Disease Eradication (ITFDE), which developed criteria for use in evaluating diseases that are considered potential candidates for eradication (Table 3.1) (Centers for Disease Control and Prevention [CDC] 1993). One important principle which has emerged clearly is that the characteristics of smallpox and the Smallpox Eradication Program, the only successful example of disease eradication so far, do not have to be replicated entirely in order for another disease to be considered potentially eradicable. Specifically, one does not have to be dealing with a viral disease using a vaccine as the intervention in order to envision eradication. In this chapter, we define eradication to mean interruption of transmission of the disease agent concerned, globally, to the extent that the disease cannot recur, even after specific control measures are ended.

We draw ten lessons from this review. Each is considered separately below.

UNDERSTAND THE NATURAL HISTORY OF THE DISEASE THOROUGHLY

Kerr (1963) has said that "to eradicate an infectious disease at minimum cost, the life history of the etiologic agent should be thoroughly known so that the eradication operations can be directed against the most vulnerable points in the chain of disease transmission." One of smallpox's most vulnerable points turned out to be its natural seasonal declines in incidence, which made control measures during periods of low incidence much more effective than the same measures implemented at other times of the year. This epidemiologic feature was fully exploited during the later stages of the smallpox eradication campaign (Fenner et al. 1988). When yellow fever eradication activities were initiated, the existence and importance of jungle yellow fever, deriving from a previously unknown nonhuman reservoir of the infection in monkeys in which transmission occurred with a vector other than *Aedes aegypti*, was not known. Had this aspect of the natural history of yellow fever been understood, it seems likely that "eradication" would not have been attempted in many areas where it was.

Knowledge of the frequency of latent or inapparent infections and the existence of any long-term carrier states can also be critical. At the beginning of the yaws campaign, for example, emphasis was placed only on the need to treat a high percentage of persons with overt disease. Only later was it realized that for every patient seen (and treated) with infectious yaws, there are about ten others with active disease and 30 more with latent infections, all of whom were liable to relapse into infectious disease after mass treatment teams departed from an area. That inadequate understanding of yaws' epidemiology was a major factor in the early failures of that campaign (Hackett and Guthe 1956). (The inability to distinguish definitively the organism or the serological response of humans to yaws from that of venereal syphilis and other closely related spirochetes which also infect humans are other features of yaws which still cause concern: how to know and prove that yaws has been eradicated?) Similarly, the high infectiousness of measles virus was underestimated in some earlier efforts to eradicate that disease (Langmuir 1970).

Continued research is necessary throughout an eradication program, both to complete knowledge on the natural history of infection (if necessary) and to monitor changes occurring as a result of interventions. Additionally, targeted research may develop highly useful tools, such as the bifurcated needle, which was a great assistance in smallpox eradication.

CONSULT WIDELY BEFORE EMBARKING ON ERADICATION

Given the global and absolute implications of eradication, the goal should not be embraced without systematic consideration of all aspects of the feasibility of eradication, and wide consultation aiming toward consensus. This consideration and consultation should include the full range of scientific feasibility and political will/popular support criteria described by the ITFDE (Table 3.1). It should also include discussions with politicians and international agencies, as well as medical and public health scientists. It is necessary is to reduce the potential risks of over-optimism/enthusiasm as well as of unwarranted skepticism. The early campaigns to eradicate hookworm and yellow fever in the Americas were reportedly initiated by the Rockefeller Foundation with only minimal advice from a few consultants.

Even wide consultation does not necessarily guarantee success, however. The same 1953 World Health Assembly (WHA) that adopted the fateful resolution to eradicate malaria globally also rejected a proposed resolution calling for the eradication of smallpox (Henderson 1987). Another benefit of wide consultation in advance is to enlist the support of all or most of the countries concerned, since at the least a regional or subregional approach is required for eradication of any disease. Failure to involve all affected countries puts whatever is gained at great risk of either being lost or requiring expensive measures to prevent reintroduction of the disease from other affected areas.

It is also important to avoid trivializing the concept of disease eradication by invoking it inappropriately or in ways that damage its credibility. As stated by the ITFDE, "care should be taken to reserve the use of the terms 'eradication' and 'elimination' only for carefully chosen diseases that have a high likelihood of being eradicated" (CDC 1993).

Although a successful eradication program is costly, a failed eradication program may be even more costly. Successful eradication requires intensive funding for a limited period. Those involved with a failing eradication program are likely to feel that a major cause of the failure is insufficient resources and consequently may request more and more resources to try to shore up the program by doing more and more of the primary intervention or adding other interventions. In addition, there is likely to be a considerable delay before it is realized that eradication is not feasible and the intensive expenditure of resources may continue for a longer period than the original eradication effort was scheduled to last.

The costs of a failed eradication program may not only be financial, however. Andrews and Langmuir (1963) believed that "if we do not succeed in experimental efforts at specific communicable disease eradication, it is almost certain that higher orders of control will be produced than would have been accomplished otherwise." By contrast, the ITFDE concluded that "if the concept of eradication is invoked against inappropriate or unattainable targets, it can again be brought into disrepute" (CDC 1993). Henderson (1987) believes, for example, that the failed malaria eradication effort had a dampening effect on other health programs: "National immunization programs were all but non-existent, sanitation schemes received little attention and the development of basic preventive services was postponed until the 'malaria eradication program could be integrated into the basic health services.'"

Sociologists have noted that the process of creating change (such as with an eradication program) consists of four stages: (1) articulate the problem; (2) show that there is a solution to the problem; (3) show that the solution works in the real world; and (4) provide leadership. The third step requires evidence from a demonstration or pilot project in a limited area or population. It provides protection against theoretical approaches that are impractical in the field under real conditions. Early efforts to eradicate hookworm from the southern U.S.A. were undertaken without such demonstrations. However, even a pilot demonstration is not foolproof: successful elimination of yellow fever in Cuba, the Panama Canal area, and Rio de Janeiro was part of the impetus behind the failed campaign to eradicate that virus from the Americas (Henderson 1987).

INITIATE SURVEILLANCE EARLY AND USE SURVEILLANCE INFORMATION TO GUIDE PROGRAM STRATEGY

Considering surveillance as "information for action" (Orenstein and Bernier 1990) it seems obvious that surveillance should be initiated at or before the beginning of eradication efforts. However, this has not always been the case. The yellow fever and hookworm campaigns suffered from lack of surveillance; in both instances surveillance was not begun until more than ten years after the eradication efforts were initiated (Cockburn 1961; Henderson 1987).

In the malaria eradication effort, initiation of surveillance was considered a part of the later activities of the "attack" phase. The result of this delay in initiating surveillance was that flaws in program strategy or execution did not become apparent as early as they should. Even when collected, surveillance information was not always used appropriately. For example, in some countries in Central America, information about the prevalence of malaria was collected on individual localities and dealt with as such. When the larger picture was considered, however, it became apparent that some localities considered free of malaria were quite close to other localities where transmission was still occurring, well within the flight range of the vector *Anopheles albimanus*.

The development of the search and containment strategy that ultimately eradicated smallpox is a classic example of the use of surveillance information to guide program strategy. Surveillance (and investigation) information indicated that smallpox did not spread rapidly over long distances but mostly to persons in a relatively easily defined zone of risk around the patient. This information then guided the decision to pursue the ring vaccination approach, especially in periods of low incidence.

Surveillance is also a key component of the dracunculiasis and polio eradication programs (Hinman et al. 1987; Richards and Hopkins 1990; Wright et al. 1991). An important related principle is to increase the quality and intensity of surveillance commensurate with the stage of the program. Whereas near-perfect surveillance is not necessary and may be neither practical nor affordable at the beginning of an eradication program, the need for near-perfect surveillance is inescapable towards the end of such a program. Surveillance also helps maintain the program's focus on *outcomes*, namely, levels of the disease, rather than on *processes*, such as numbers of services provided or of persons trained, vaccinated, or treated. This facilitates adjusting activities as necessary in order to reduce the disease, rather than being misled by high numbers of people reached. One senior malaria eradication official said that "the *science* of malaria control . . . was almost overnight converted to the rather simplistic *technology* of malaria eradication . . . ." (Jeffery 1976).

ERADICATION PROGRAMS REQUIRE A
VERTICAL APPROACH

By "vertical approach," we mean application of sound management principles; having a clear goal; proper training, supply, supervision, and feedback; not a separate cadre of full-time workers. There is long-standing tension between those who advocate specific disease-control (or eradication) approaches and those who feel that nothing should be done unless it advances the overall provision of comprehensive health care. We believe that targeted disease control or eradication programs "can both complement and supplement the general health services in the task of ensuring better health for the people" (WHO 1965). In that sense we tend to agree with Waddy (1956), who wrote (after many years' experience in Ghana): "the forces available to combat rural ill-health are enthusiastic but small. They should not be dissipated on too many unattainable objectives, but concentrated ruthlessly on those that can be achieved, and which careful forethought considers will do the most good."

It is certainly true that at the periphery, human resources are so limited that many or most field workers appropriately carry out more than one function. In order to achieve a specific (and absolute) goal such as disease eradication, however, it is necessary to have a small central core of staff who are specifically charged with achieving the goal. Otherwise, compromises are likely to be made which will jeopardize its achievement. E.H. Hinman (1963) stated "there must be a centralized *direction* of the campaign, but decentralized *execution* of it."

The manifest advantage of an eradication campaign, namely, being able to amortize the costs of the campaign indefinitely, with no further need for disease control expenditures, comes at the price of a higher cost to be paid up-front. That higher cost includes the need to focus on the disease to be eradicated. This is a fundamental difference between a control program and an eradication program.

Various authors have described the unique need for eradication programs to take an absolutist view and be run in an authoritarian style in order to be successful. Perhaps the most extreme manifestation of this is encapsulated in the following quote from Soper (1965, pp. 860–861):

> Once organized, meticulous administration seems logical and simple and it belied the difficulties suffered in its development. Unavoidably, such administration was criticized at times by someone who overlooked the serious responsibility of the Yellow Fever Service. The press in Niteroi once violently attacked the Service for dismissing an inspector because he had not been killed the day before. The inspector's itinerary required him to spend much of the same morning each week in the arsenal across Guanabara Bay from Rio de Janeiro. On the morning of one scheduled visit, the arsenal was destroyed by an explosion and every one on the premises perished. The press insisted that the Yellow Fever Service should have rejoiced over the inspector's escape rather than penalize him for dereliction in performance of his duty.

Eradication programs are often discussed using military terms and, in fact, some of the earliest successful local/regional eradication efforts were carried out by the military (e.g., yellow fever in Cuba by Gorgas and the U.S. Army). E.H. Hinman (1963) has described the need for "an unusual degree of autonomy" for eradication programs, including "flexibility in hiring and firing employees," etc. However, this degree of autonomy, if accompanied by total separation from other health activities, can lead to resentment from other health workers and diminish the cooperation needed to achieve the goal.

Key to implementing a successful eradication program is to ensure good supervision, training, supply, and regular feedback to the peripheral health workers concerned. It is necessary to assure that staff are always kept up-to-date about program developments (both positive and negative) and given refresher training as new techniques are implemented or situations change. That is how the dracunculiasis eradication program has developed superb surveillance and implementation in some of the poorest regions of Africa (and many other programs have not), even though many of the workers in the Guinea worm eradication program are village volunteers, or multi-purpose health workers who have not received similar support for their other broad responsibilities. Monitoring of a few key indices which are directly related to the eradication objective is also important.

REMAIN OPEN MINDED AND FLEXIBLE; EXPECT THE UNEXPECTED

Rigorous adherence to principle should not blind one to new information or changing circumstances. When the smallpox eradication program was originally launched it was felt that near-universal vaccination ($\geq 80\%$) would be necessary to achieve eradication. However, a vaccine shortage necessitated developing priorities as to who should receive vaccine and this led to the development of the "ring vaccination" approach (also called search and containment) in which only those at imminent risk of exposure were targeted. Application of this approach led to eradication of smallpox in several countries where far fewer than 80% of the population had been vaccinated (Fenner et al. 1988).

By contrast, the initial success in eliminating malaria opened up many areas to rapid agricultural development which led to major influxes of new residents to those areas and called for a degree of flexibility which often was not present (A.R. Hinman 1984). Although a high degree of uniformity is needed, successful eradication will almost certainly require adaptation to local circumstances rather than a "one size fits all" approach. Collins and Paskewitz (1995) said, "We must remember the lesson of the now abandoned global malaria eradication campaign: Malaria cannot be dealt with as a single and uniform worldwide problem, susceptible to one global control strategy."

It is not possible to predict exactly *what* unexpected events will occur but it is possible to predict that such events will occur. It is wise to anticipate what kinds of things might go wrong and be prepared to deal with them, insofar as possible. Continuing research is needed to aid in "identifying and overcoming ecological obstacles to eradication that are encountered" (Kerr 1963). Operational research is also important in maintaining flexibility and the ability to respond to changing circumstances, surveillance data, other new information, etc. Modeling may help in anticipating changes in epidemiology of disease during the course of the program.

The Guinea worm eradication program changed its initial strategy of improving rural water supply as the main intervention (during the International Drinking Water Supply and Sanitation Decade) to the faster and less expensive interventions of health education and use of cloth filters based on experience gathered during the campaign (Hopkins and Ruiz-Tiben 1991).

SOME COUNTRIES WILL NEED MORE HELP THAN OTHERS

Diseases slated for eradication are likely to be most concentrated in developing countries which have the fewest resources to devote to the effort. Consequently, both technical and financial support from external donors may be critical. This may be particularly true if commodities such as a vaccine (or insecticide) have to be purchased in international markets using hard currency. Nonetheless, when total program costs are examined, the endemic countries clearly shoulder the major burden, primarily through the costs of local personnel. For example, in the current polio eradication program, donors such as Rotary International are providing massive support (US$ 400 million from Rotary alone over the course of the program), but more than two-thirds of total program costs are still estimated to be borne by host countries. A similar estimate was made for the smallpox eradication program. Additionally, there may be ways (such as the creation of "revolving funds") in which the host country can use local currency to offset donor expenditures within the country, freeing up the donor's hard currency to be used for purchasing the commodities. Since some of these donor expenditures might not have been slated for the eradication program, this may further increase the proportion of total costs borne by the host country, and donors should be sensitive to this possibility.

One must be prepared to help countries where the targeted disease is not a high national priority, e.g., because its incidence or mortality rate is low. This was the case in East Africa with smallpox, where the strain of smallpox virus was fatal in less than 1% of infected persons. More recently, it is the case in Cameroon and Kenya, where Guinea worm disease is a minor problem in a remote corner of the country. Yet these countries, too, must eliminate the disease if the regional effort is to succeed. One must also recognize the special self-interest in some countries. For example, one advantage for the United States in fostering eradication of smallpox, polio, and measles abroad is that it was and is a very cost-effective way of protecting its own citizens at home. Cockburn (1961) said:

Great difficulty arises in areas where an infection of global or continental significance is of no particular public health importance locally. It is difficult to persuade a community to put up the funds and make the effort required for something that causes little local inconvenience. For example, a few countries joined in malaria eradication only after some hesitation; for them, malaria was simply not a public health problem, and there was no public pressure to organize expensive measures to benefit neighboring countries.

COORDINATION OF EXTERNAL DONORS IS ESSENTIAL

An essential feature of the polio eradication program has been the creation of donor coordinating committees at national and regional levels. This is true partly because of the need to deal with the differing mandates of different agencies which are seeking to collaborate on a common objective. These committees can help assure that all legitimate needs are met and that duplication of efforts (and donations) does not occur. Additionally, such committees serve a major role in increasing donor "ownership" of the program and enthusiasm toward it. Many international donors (such as Rotary International) may have local chapters which, if involved, can provide important additional assistance, physical, financial, and political. In the Guinea worm eradication program donor coordination is achieved during quarterly or semi-annual interagency coordination meetings and during annual program reviews of individual programs.

POLITICAL COMMITMENTS FROM ALL LEVELS
ARE ESSENTIAL

Political will must be manifested in order for eradication to succeed. Achieving the necessary level of political will requires political skill. An important feature of the polio eradication program has been enlisting the support of national leaders in the campaign. For example, Presidents, Prime Ministers, and First Ladies have all been highly visible administering oral polio vaccine on National Immunization Days (NIDs). To remove partisan flavor from political support, efforts should be made to enlist support from the opposition as well as the party in power. It has even been possible, in both Central America and Africa, to get leaders of warring factions to declare a cease-fire in order to carry out NIDs and protect all children in the country. Similarly, a four-month cease-fire was negotiated in Sudan to permit Guinea worm eradication activities to take place. The need for high-level political commitment is just as great at the local and international level. The former president of the United States, Jimmy Carter, and the former head of state of Mali, General Amadou Toumani Toure, have been important figures in stimulating high-level support within individual countries for Guinea worm eradication. Similar high-level involvement also characterized the smallpox eradication program. Political commitments may also be stimulated by appropriate use of data, e.g., contrasting the level of a particular disease in an area/country with its level in another (neighboring) area/country.

Just as it is essential to involve political leaders, it is essential to involve the general public in all phases of the program and keep them informed. Community members know their communities and what will work or not work. In addition, they are much more likely to be genuinely supportive of an eradication program if they feel they have had a role in creating and implementing it. Consequently, involving them from the earliest phases of a program is good sense as well as good politics. By the same token it is essential to keep the public fully informed about program developments, both positive and negative. The key to ultimate success is strong community partnerships.

INSPIRE ENTHUSIASM, BUT DON'T DECLARE SUCCESS PREMATURELY

Strong leadership is critical to the success of eradication. It is essential for leaders to be enthusiastic in order to inspire their staff. However, although it is appropriate to be pleased with progress, it is important to remain vigilant and remember that the last cases (by definition) are going to be the hardest and costliest to prevent. As Cockburn (1961) wrote:

> In a country where conditions favor the parasite, the elimination of this last trace of the infection can be extremely troublesome; yet until it has been accomplished, the campaign will not be a success. If the operating procedures are stopped prematurely, the infection will return, and either the program will have to be recommenced or else all the effort will have been wasted.

This has occurred, for example, with malaria (in Sri Lanka) and yaws (in Haiti and Ghana). It is essential to focus on how much remains to be accomplished rather than enjoying how much has been done. Although uncomfortable, it may be useful to have a professional skeptic who will constantly be looking for things that are *not* going well and raising questions about what remains to be done.

A related problem is to maintain enthusiasm among program staff as the disease becomes less frequent and harder to find. According to Soper (1965):

> In control, one may measure progress from the high point on the curve of incidence downward, ie, what has been done; in eradication one measures always from the base line of the chart upward, ie, what remains to be done. In control, one tends to lose interest in a disease at the point where, in eradication, many times, the greatest difficulties are encountered.

In considering the smallpox eradication program in India, Brilliant (1985) described the "realm of the final inch":

> Many programs lose momentum and are prematurely declared to be successful .... The realm of the final inch, the meticulous attention to detail for a two-year period of painstaking and sometimes unrewarding surveillance, is one of the most revealing aspects of the smallpox programs .... The use of outside evaluators and the importance given to outside evaluation was another incentive to keep up high standards of work.

The smallpox program, the Guinea worm program, and the polio eradication program have all used cash rewards as incentives to maintain the degree of surveillance needed in the final stages of eradication.

There is also a risk of losing financial, political, and managerial support before the job is done if success is declared prematurely. One of the mistakes of the yaws eradication effort was premature "integration" of control measures into the general health services of countries, when those general health services were unable to continue the levels of surveillance and follow up which were still required. Haiti reduced the level of reported yaws from 45,356 cases in 1949 to about 400 cases in 1953 (Cockburn 1961); Ghana and other countries achieved similarly spectacular results (Agadzie et al. 1985), which were lost as incidence of the disease rose again after responsibility for surveillance and control passed from specialized teams to the general health services, which were still too weak to support them.

Eradication programs have been important sources of well-trained and highly motivated staff for other health programs. Because of this, on occasion eradication staff have been transferred to other programs to their benefit but at some risk to the successful completion of eradication. Because of the close interrelationship of eradication programs and general health services, eradication programs should explicitly address their impact on general health services and efforts should be made to maximize the effectiveness of both the short-term (eradication) and long-term (overall health service development) programs.

SET A SPECIFIC TARGET DATE FOR ERADICATION

Despite previous WHA resolutions, the smallpox eradication program floundered until 1966, when the target was established to achieve eradication within 10 years, even though the target date was not included in the 1966 WHA resolution. The establishment of a target date of 1995 for Guinea worm eradication by African ministers of health (in 1988) and the WHA (in 1991) was a powerful stimulus to the program. Similarly, the establishment in 1985 (by the ministers of health of the Americas) of a 1990 target date for polio eradication from the Western Hemisphere was essential to the success of the program. The fact that the smallpox target was ten months late in achievement and the polio target was eight months late was inconsequential — what was important was to focus the campaign for health authorities and workers and highlight the time-limited nature of the program for potential donors.

The target date chosen is dependent on the technology and natural history of the disease. From a practical point of view, a target date much greater than ten years in the future may not be able to inspire and sustain the enthusiasm necessary for the task.

Urgency is implicit in an eradication program. Not only is there the issue of the duration of extra effort needed, but two other factors make achievement of the goal urgent: 1) the all-or-none nature of the goal, which means that all countries remain at risk so long as any country remains infected, and 2) the unpredictability of human behavior, which means that civil or military disruption in any of the areas concerned can jeopardize the successful conclusion of the program. Consideration of the criteria for certification of eradication should begin at the earliest stages of the program.

CONCLUSION

A final lesson, which may seem self-evident, is that *eradication of some diseases is possible, but it is not easy.* The fact that smallpox was eradicated demonstrates that it is possible. The difficulties encountered in the unsuccessful programs (as well as in the smallpox, dracunculiasis, and polio programs) make it clear that it is not easy. The fact that it is difficult, however, should not prevent consideration of the possibility, since the benefits of eradication are eternal, whereas the effort is time-limited. Eradication is the ultimate in communicable disease control and in sustainability.

REFERENCES

Agadzie, V.K., Y. Aboagye-Atta, J.W. Nelson, D.R. Hopkins, and P.L. Perine. 1985. Yaws in Ghana. *Rev. Infec. Dis.* **7(2)**:S233–S236.

Andrews, J.M., and A.D. Langmuir. 1963. The philosophy of disease eradication. *Am. J. Pub. Hlth.* **53**:1–6.

Brilliant, L. 1985. The Management of Smallpox Eradication in India. Ann Arbor: Univ. of Michigan Press.

CDC (Centers for Disease Control and Prevention). 1993. Recommendations of the International Task Force for Disease Eradication. *Morbid. Mortal. Wkly. Rep.* **42 (RR–16)**:1–38.

Cockburn, T.A. 1961. Eradication of infectious diseases. *Science* **133**:1050–1058.

Collins, F.H., and S.M. Paskewitz. 1995. Malaria: Current and future prospects for control. *Ann. Rev. Entomol.* **40**:195–219.

Fenner, F., D.A. Henderson, I. Arita, Z. Jezek, and I.D. Ladnyi. 1988. Smallpox and Its Eradication. Geneva: WHO.

Hackett, C.J., and T. Guthe. 1956. Some important aspects of yaws eradication. *Bull. WHO* **15**:869–896.

Henderson, D.A. 1987. Eradication: Pitfalls and Promise. The Eighth Joseph Mountin Lecture, delivered at the Centers for Disease Control and Prevention.

Hinman, A.R. 1984. Prospects for disease eradication or elimination. *NY St. J. Med.* **84**:502–506.

Hinman, A.R., W.H. Foege, C.A. de Quadros, P.A. Patriarca, W.A. Orenstein, and E.W. Brink. 1987. The case for global eradication of poliomyelitis. *Bull. WHO* **65**:835–840.

Hinman, E.H. 1963. Current status of eradication of infectious diseases. *Trans. Coll. Phys. Phila.* **80**:855–869.

Hopkins, D.R., and E. Ruiz-Tiben. 1991. Strategies for dracunculiasis eradication. *Bull. WHO* **69**:533–540.

Jeffery, G.M. 1976. Malaria control in the twentieth century. *Am. J. Trop. Med. Hyg.* **25**:361–371.

Kerr, J.A. 1963. Lessons to be learned from failures to eradicate. *Am. J. Pub. Hlth.* **53**:27–30.

Langmuir, A.D. 1970. Prospects for eradication of viral diseases by immunization. In: Proc. Intl. Conf. on the Application of Vaccines against Viral, Rickettsial, and Bacterial Diseases of Man. Washington, D.C: Pan American Health Organization.

Orenstein, W.A., and R.H. Bernier. 1990. Surveillance: Information for action. *Pediatr. Clin. N. Am.* **37**:709–734.

Richards, F., Jr., and D.R. Hopkins. 1990. Surveillance: The foundation for control and elimination of dracunculiasis in Africa. *Intl. J. Epidemiol.* **18**:934–943.

Soper, F.L. 1965. Rehabilitation of the eradication concept in prevention of communicable diseases. *Pub. Hlth. Rep.* **80**:855–869.

Waddy, B.B. 1956. Organization and work of the Gold Coast Medical Field Units. *Trans. Roy. Soc. Trop. Med. Hyg.* **50**:313–336.

WHO (World Health Organization). 1965. Integration of mass campaigns against specific diseases into general health services. Report of a WHO Study Group. WHO Technical Report Series No. 294. Geneva: WHO.

Wright, P.F., R.J. Kim-Farley, C.A. de Quadros, S.E. Robertson, R.M.C.N. Scott, N.A. Ward, and R.H. Henderson. 1991. Strategies for the global eradication of poliomyelitis by the year 2000. *New Engl. J. Med.* **325**:1774–1779.

4

The Role of Mathematical Models in Eradication of Infectious Disease

G.F. MEDLEY, D.J. NOKES, and W.J. EDMUNDS

Dept. of Biological Sciences, University of Warwick, Coventry, CV4 7AL, U.K.

ABSTRACT

Mathematical models of transmission dynamics of infectious disease are becoming increasingly seen as useful tools to aid in the design of control programs. This is partly because they provide insight into inherently nonlinear processes, but also, and perhaps more importantly, because they act as a bridge between public health and health economics. However, although models produce results valuable to the design of control programs against endemic infections, they are underdeveloped with respect to control of outbreaks and assessment of risks of reintroduced diseases into populations from which they were eliminated.

INTRODUCTION

In this chapter we provide a synopsis of the role of mathematical models in the design of cost-effective control programs against infectious diseases. These control programs may lead to elimination (from specified geographical regions) or eradication (global extinction), but their aims may, or may not, be cost-effective, depending on how economic costs are viewed. It is perhaps unwise to begin a program with eradication as a fixed goal. Eradication is more likely recognized as a feasible option when infection and disease are fairly tightly controlled, and when elimination has been achieved in large geographic areas.

Typically, although not exclusively (e.g., polio in Central and South America), the pattern is for developed countries to control and eliminate first, providing the impetus for eradication by elimination in developing countries. The effort to eradicate is thus developed from experience in control and elimination, and many of the lessons of how to control have been learnt at this point. Consequently, at first sight, transmission dynamic models will play a small role in development of eradication strategies, as the

The Eradication of Infectious Diseases
Edited by W.R. Dowdle and D.R. Hopkins © 1998 John Wiley and Sons Ltd.

control methodology will be understood and the principal concerns will be economic and logistic. Note that we do not discuss the use of mathematical models in terms of operational and logistical analyses, but confine ourselves to models of purely biological processes.

Control of infection must be seen as the first step in eradication. As we discuss, mathematical models are a natural tool to aid development of control strategies. They provide considerable insight into what processes govern the transmission of infection and the development of subsequent disease, and the effect of different control strategies. This insight can lead to classification of infections into those that may possibly be eradicated (and the expected time scale of eradication) and those infections for which eradication is not currently feasible. For the latter category, it is possible to point to the barriers preventing eradication and so develop research agendas for development of appropriate tools. Once control has been successfully achieved, a new set of problems emerge, namely, the ascertainment of risk of and prevention of outbreaks.

We begin a brief discussion of the role of mathematical modeling generally. We emphasize that mathematical modeling should be viewed as any other scientific procedure (such as polymerase chain reaction); it can serve some purposes very well, and its existence opens the possibilities of new goals, but, as with all techniques, there are limitations and misuses that should be understood if the technique is to be employed effectively. We then consider some of the complications of modeling, in particular heterogeneities that must be considered with models, and the issue of the perspective of the model. A complete discussion of the results of modeling is beyond the scope of this chapter, but we point out some of the classifications that are evident, before discussing the role of models during the process of control, during eradication and afterwards.

An Ecological Aside

The theory of infectious disease control, and its mathematical models, comes from population biology, just as diagnostic methods come from biochemistry. The control of infectious agents and the conservation of biological diversity are essentially the same subject, but with opposite aims. It should be noted in any book on the eradication of infectious disease that many of the world's ecologists are working hard not to eradicate species. We believe it to be a serious ethical question as to whether infectious agents should be exterminated, but as public opinion does not mount campaigns to "Save the polio virus" in the same way as "Save the whale," we choose to ignore these arguments here.

THE NECESSITY FOR MATHEMATICAL MODELS

In this section we address the arguments as to why mathematical models are necessary by presenting the essential features of infectious disease epidemiology, and then point out, generally, what can and cannot be achieved with these tools.

Infectious Disease Epidemiology

Infectious disease is fundamentally different from noninfectious disease in that the risks of disease to an individual are intrinsically linked to the risk to others in the population: incidence is a function of prevalence. For noninfectious disease, there is no such connection — an individual developing heart disease does not increase the risk of other individuals in the population developing heart disease. Conversely, an individual who is infected with a pathogen *does* increase the risk of others contracting the infection. The corollary is that protection of an individual from infection reduces the risk of infection of other individuals, so that any intervention preventing infection in a proportion of individuals has immediate benefits for those individuals at whom the intervention was not targeted or was not given. This link between incidence and prevalence has two principal consequences.

First, that mathematical models of infection (and its control) must be based within communities or populations. Much of the research on cost-effectiveness of vaccination programs employ a cohort model structure which implicitly assumes that the total risk of infection in a population of 1000 people is 1000 times the risk to a single individual, which is clearly not true (see, e.g., Margolis et al. 1995; Edmunds et al. 1996b, and submitted). Immunizing 999 of a (closed) population of 1000 also protects the unvaccinated person.

Consequently, infectious disease requires mathematical tools that are nonlinear. This is because biological populations are controlled by processes that are nonlinear. For example, doubling the number of vaccine dose given or halving the density of vectors will not result in halving of disease incidence. Parasites (including microparasites) are held at endemic levels by density-dependent constraints. Reducing the incidence or prevalence of infection reduces the effect of the constraints, which acts to mitigate against the intervention employed.

Second, policies optimized for the individuals within a population are not necessarily the best for the whole population. Vaccination provides a good example, where given that vaccination carries some small risk itself, the optimum for any individual is for the rest of the population to be vaccinated while remaining unvaccinated herself. This type of conflict is common to economics and environmental management, and is further discussed in Medley (1996).

Additionally, infectious disease is unique in that the etiological agent is a biological entity under genetic control that is subject to the same rules of adaption and selection as all other organisms. Consequently, any control policy adopted will impose selective pressure, which may result in the selection of strains of a pathogen with specific changes that overcome or mitigate the control policy. This is seen most dramatically in terms of development of drug resistance. However, there is also the possibility of antigenic changes to circumvent immunity induced by vaccination (McLean 1995).

Infection and Disease

Transmission dynamic models clearly show the distinction between infection and disease. It is infection that must be modeled directly, as it is the chain of infection that maintains the parasite in the host population. In this context, modeling the disease requires knowledge about what factors determine which individuals will develop disease given that they are infected (Edmunds, Medley et al. 1997). These factors might include infectious dose, nutrition, and genetics. These factors are not strictly necessary in attempting to eradicate infection and are a relatively uncommon inclusion in mathematical models of infection dynamics. This distinction does raise the question of whether the eradication of disease is possible or advisable without the eradication of infection.

What Mathematical Models Can Do

For modelers, the principal role of models is to provide a framework within which all aspects (individual, population, national) and different levels (molecular, immunological, epidemiological, and economic) can be combined. This framework, or rather the holes in it when under construction, provide a research agenda. The model also provides a natural link between data and hypothesis. Comparison between model outcomes and between model results and observation allows a real development of understanding of the importance of different processes, and it is this aspect that allows for the design of cost-effective control strategies.

Prediction is usually the nonmodeler's view of the principal role. If you require quantitative predictions then models are required. Models can and do fulfill this role, but rarely are models to be considered complete or comprehensive enough to predict quantitatively beyond the short term.

It is also important to note that mathematical models themselves can be a very cost-effective means of evaluation of control programs. They lead to less reliance on large-scale field trials, which may be expensive both financially and in terms of health costs. Careful modeling also guides the scope and parameter ranges over which trials are conducted. Obviously, models are the only way in which eradication programs can be evaluated.

What Mathematical Models Cannot Do

The obvious point is that models cannot ask questions but can only provide answers to specific questions. It is tempting to think that by constructing a model, the process of control and eradication is simply a matter of obeying the instructions issued by the model. Models, however, are tools to aid design and will only do so if they are used as an integral part of the process managing the interventions.

MODEL STRUCTURES

Fundamental to the study of simple models (i.e., those without complicating heterogeneity) is the concept of the basic reproduction number, R_0. This parameter measures the intrinsic ability of a parasite to invade and persist in specified host populations

(Anderson and May 1991). It comprises aspects of the three basic factors determining the epidemiology of an infectious disease: the natural history of infection (especially the duration of infectiousness), the route of transmission and the environment/behavior of the population (the important aspects of which are determined by the route of transmission). However, simple models fail to include complicating factors (such as differences between individuals, time-dependent changes, factors external to the "closed" population) that are thought or known to be important.

Throughout applied mathematical modeling there is a compromise to be drawn between complexity and usefulness. The real world is hopelessly complicated, and the object of models is to reduce the complexity to a level that is both comprehensible and tractable. Too much complexity leads to model output that may be as incomprehensible as the real world. From this viewpoint, models are better developed with increasing complexity until either the model is sufficiently accurate to answer the question being addressed, or until available data to estimate parameters and validate model output is exhausted. The art of model development is to include sufficient complexity to make the model valuable, but simple enough to understand, which necessarily requires that an understanding is developed of the importance of different processes in determining model behavior.

Models should not be regarded as providing *the answer,* but rather should be regarded as tools to increase understanding, highlight important processes, and find potential hypotheses to explain observed phenomena. Mathematics provides the tools to analyze models in the same way as biochemistry provides the tools to analyze biological specimens. Consequently, any model, such as ill-defined computer simulations, that do not specify the mathematics they are using should be regarded suspiciously. Although there is some (heated) debate within modeling communities over "mathematical" and "simulation" approaches (see, e.g., Habbema et al. 1996 and the following discussion), this is largely irrelevant to application as long as the assumptions and techniques are clearly defined. The key aspect, to our mind, is that the modeling be presented as repeatable science rather than as a "black box."

Happily, experience suggests that the results of the simplest models can be found in more complex models, and that they can reproduce many observed phenomena. Thus, the simplest models of a close contact, childhood virus are able to reproduce periodic epidemics, realistic age-seroprevalence and epidemic patterns as well as herd immunity.

Heterogeneities

The principal complexity complicating model structures is heterogeneity, both between individuals (in terms of risk of infection from other members of the population), and in pathogens (especially in terms of antigenic variation). This is an area of active research in infectious disease epidemiology that is focused on a variety of potentially important problems, such as: how can sexual behavior networks be characterized, and why are only four serotypes of rotavirus commonly found in humans? These questions may be of considerable importance in determining the possibility of eradication. However, given that control must be achieved before eradication is considered, these questions may be better considered as reflecting current concerns in control rather than eradication.

One of the most ubiquitous of heterogeneities is variability with respect to age. The age of an individual determines the rate (and type) of contact with other individuals (of different ages) in a population, and so determines the risk of infection from other individuals (of different ages) (Edmunds, O'Callaghan et al. 1997). For example, children of early school age are likely to have greater contact with others of the same age than those 10–15 yrs older, and will not generally be at risk of contracting sexually transmitted infections. An important characteristic of age is that all individuals experience (or have the potential to experience) all ages. Age is also important because of its relationship to the probability of developing disease on infection for a variety of pathogen species. Control generally increases the average of infection in those individuals not protected and may result in a shift in the age-related pattern of disease observed, or even increase the total amount of disease. Hepatitus B (HBV) provides an interesting example in which increasing average age at infection can have both positive and negative public health benefits (Edmunds et al. 1996c).

Perspective

Of central importance in using mathematical models correctly is to define the perspective within which the model sits, in the same way as economic models sit within specified perspectives. A transmission dynamic model must take a population (rather than individual) perspective if it is to reflect infectious disease epidemiology accurately. Then the question becomes: which population? The potential range of population sizes could be from single villages to global. For all but global models, there are effects that occur outside the population being modeled. For instance, the immunization rate in one city influences the rate of infection in a neighboring city, or the rate of immunization on one birth cohort influences the rate of infection in other birth cohorts. These additional effects are known as externalities in economic terms. As the scope of a model increases, the number and complexity of potential externalities decrease, but the number and complexity of internal heterogeneities increases. Thus, any model is a compromise between complexity and completeness.

As a specific example, consider the case of a directly transmitted microparasite infection. Models for homogeneous and heterogeneous transmission have been widely used to investigate the impact of vaccination policies (e.g., Anderson and May 1984). While the inclusion of age-related heterogeneity and limited spatial heterogeneity have been accomplished in such models with useful results, the general predictive value of any model decreases as heterogeneity increases (due to inclusion of more parameters). Thus, models used to investigate vaccination policies for rubella have largely been at the level of a small town, as they have ignored spatial factors. At this level, all of the parameters are, to lesser or greater extent, measurable or inferable from independent data. The use of such models for design of national vaccination strategies must assume that the national situation can be considered as a collection of independent small towns. The construction of a national model proper would require estimates of the rates of transmission between different towns and cities. These estimates are not achievable directly, so the model would have to include a degree of "guesswork" and assumption to define all model parameters. In reality, the models developed thus far would appear to be useful and accurate tools, suggesting that, for example, spatial patterns are secondary in importance to age-related mixing patterns for determining national vaccination policy against endemic infections such as measles. However, when control is achieved, and outbreak prevention is important, spatial factors are likely to be more important.

By definition, a vaccination policy rests at a supra-individual level, usually national. Consequently, within a model to be used to design national vaccination policy, those aspects outside of the national body's direct control must be considered as externalities. This includes, most importantly, the continual introduction of the infectious agent into a population. In much of Western Europe and North America, measles has become essentially *eliminated*; in the United Kingdom, overall annual incidence has been reduced to very low levels with most of the infections traceable to imported cases. Consequently, the risk of infection is, without considering externalities, zero, or very nearly zero. Within a model this continual importation of infection would have to be included as a constant immigration of infectious individuals, with no guidance as to when such immigration would cease, i.e., when *global eradication* occurs. As this eventuality is outside of the immediate national jurisdiction, any economic study of a vaccination program at the national level will have to assume continual vaccination, with no time of cessation. Global eradication cannot be included in national models of vaccination program design. Global eradication can only be considered in models of global immunization programs, which must by necessity deal with heterogeneities on a worldwide scale. These issues are discussed more by Edmunds, Medley, and Nokes (submitted).

Externalities also exist in the biological processes. For example, animal hosts frequently play a role as reservoir hosts, and eradication of, for example, human rabies or schistosomiasis would require eradication in all hosts.

THE LIKELIHOOD OF ERADICATION

It is undoubtedly true that there is a spectrum with regard to the potential for eradication. Mathematical modeling can be used fruitfully to determine where specific infectious diseases sit on the scale with current technologies. Those infections that are potentially possible to eradicate include pathogens that have a relatively low basic reproduction number, for example, a slower growth rate in epidemic situations (relative to infections with similar generation times). Generally, infections with high basic reproduction numbers are more difficult to eradicate. However, the basic reproduction number does not include a number of factors that determine eradication potential, which are now discussed.

Antigenic Variation

Vaccines are notoriously difficult to develop for infections that display a large population genetic variation, chiefly because antigenic changes are already existent, probably to circumvent the immunity developed to natural infection. In fact, it is salient to consider that those infections for which eradication is probable by vaccination are those infections that are generally monotypic, close contact transmitted, highly contagious viruses. These viruses would appear to have been selected for high transmission in large populations rather than survival in small communities, and are thus vulnerable to reduction in the size of the susceptible population.

In monotypic viruses such as measles, the idea of critical community size is important (Keeling and Grenfell 1997). Where the natural history of the infection is such that individuals are infected once, and then become immune, so-called SIR (susceptible-infectious-resistant) or SEIR (susceptible-exposed-infectious-resistant) infections, the transmission dynamics are such that there is a community size below which the infection is likely to become extinct due to the rate of supply of susceptible individuals (from births). For measles, theoretical and empirical observations suggest this community size is about 300,000 individuals. This represents the size of population for which elimination is a guaranteed natural phenomena. All that is required is to ensure that infection is not introduced into this population, and, if it is, it will produce an epidemic and become eliminated again. The phenomenon demonstrates that SIR infections are essentially easier to eradicate because of their dependence on a continual supply of susceptibles via birth. This supply can be curtailed by vaccination.

Those infections for which individuals do not generate life-long immunity and where individuals become susceptible again after primary infection, so-called SIS (susceptible-infectious-susceptible) infections, do not demonstrate fade out, neither theoretical nor empirically, and are consequently much more difficult to eradicate. Examples include respiratory syncytial virus (RSV), rotavirus, and most sexually transmitted infections. Essentially, the whole population constitutes susceptibles. Additionally, the ability to reinfect individuals usually derives from antigenic diversity, thus making the development of vaccines more difficult.

Time Scales

For microparasites, the natural time scale of the transmission dynamics is determined by the length of the period between infection and immunity (the generation time). Short, acute infections show rapid epidemics, and because of the antagonism with demographic time scales, tend to show periodic oscillations in incidence. Control of transmission and infection in this case has immediate effects on the incidence of disease. The introduction of vaccination against measles and polio show immediate effects on transmission. Infections with longer infectious periods are dynamically slower, and control will necessarily change incidence on a longer time scale. HBV, with a carrier state of typically many decades duration, will require many decades of immunization to eradicate (Edmunds et al. 1996b; Williams et al. 1996). Only if treatment is developed to cure carriage (and so curtail the infectious period) can HBV be eradicated within a shorter time scale.

Transmission Heterogeneity and Immuno-modulation

Recent theoretical developments (Dushoff 1996; Gubbins and Gilligan, unpublished manuscript) have introduced the idea that the abilities of a pathogen to invade (cause an epidemic) and persist (become endemic) in a population are dependent on the prevalence of infection. Dushoff proposes that if incidence increases more than linearly with prevalence, then the threshold for an epidemic depends on the size of the initial introduction. In other words, the presence of the pathogen alters its environment (i.e., the host population) in such a way that it is more conducive to the pathogen. A biological mechanism that could generate such a phenomenon would be immunological tolerance induced by continual exposure. Removal of the parasite would result in a decrease in tolerance, so that the pathogen would be unable to reinvade the same population. In terms of design of control programs, this effect is similar to that of the breakpoint introduced for dioecious helminths (Anderson and May 1991). Whether these effects are important remains to be seen. They do, however, illustrate that understanding of elemental processes is still developing.

TOWARDS ERADICATION

In this section we briefly show how models have informed the design of control strategies. As an infectious disease is increasingly controlled, and eradication becomes a feasible goal, the requirements of models change. In particular, endemic diseases become sporadic and epidemic, and the spectrum (particularly by age) of individuals infected changes. Attention turns increasingly towards the quantification of risk of epidemics and their mitigation. This is shown up starkly when considering the emergence of previously unrecognized diseases or the reemergence of pathogens that were considered controlled.

Optimum Control Design

There are many examples where models have helped design control programs. We will not attempt an exhaustive list but provide some examples. In the case of vaccination, models have been used to determine the minimum coverage rate required in continuous mass vaccination in order to eliminate infection (Anderson and May 1991). Models have addressed the questions of age of vaccination (Anderson and May 1991), spatial patterns (Anderson and May 1984), choice of vaccine (Nokes and Anderson 1990), and requirements for booster doses (Edmunds et al. 1996c). Similar results are appearing for the design of pulse vaccination programs (Nokes and Swinton 1997).

In terms of mass chemotherapy against helminth infections, results show that it is more cost-effective to treat as many people as possible in each round of treatment, rather than increase the frequency of treatment (Guyatt et al. 1995). This is largely because of the effect of treatment on those untreated, a process that reappears throughout infectious disease epidemiology.

In reality, optimization for eradication is difficult. Within any model, there must be constraints preventing eradication (eradication in models is easy!). These can either be simply stated (e.g., vaccination coverage can never be more than 50%), or the context can be shifted to include economic processes and asking optimization questions: cost-effectiveness. As eradication follows control, it usually requires that there is an intervention effort well beyond the optimum that would be found from any modeling framework.

From Endemic to Epidemic

Successful control programs reduce incidence of infection to levels well below the endemic level. For vaccination programs, when the majority of individuals are vaccinated, the level of immunity is sufficient to prevent widespread epidemics on a national scale. The pattern of, e.g., measles changes from that of endemic, with almost all children becoming infected by the age of ten years, to that of relatively isolated outbreaks (i.e., localized and limited epidemics). Given that older individuals born during the period immediately after the introduction of vaccination are less likely to have been infected (and are therefore more likely to be susceptible to infection), and that antibody titers wane (Gay 1996) with age (and time since infection/vaccination), what infection does occur will increasingly be recognized in older individuals. Mass infant vaccination is likely to change a universal, childhood viral infection into a sporadic infection of older individuals.

This implies that the current models are destined to be replaced by frameworks that are directed towards the prediction and modeling of outbreaks. One of the essential differences between modeling endemic, common infections and sporadic, limited infections is that in the latter stochastic, or chance, effects are important, and, indeed, may predominate in determining the pattern of infection and disease. While there is considerable theoretical understanding of outbreaks/epidemics, there has been relatively little research into the direct application of this theory, and there is consequently little consistency in policies at the national level (or lower) to control outbreaks of any infection. This is partly because of the stochastic nature of any model output, which must be in terms of risks.

The scale of an epidemic resulting from reintroduction of a disease into a population from which it has been eliminated depends on the epidemiological characteristics of the pathogen, but also on host population factors. These host factors will usually be different from those that are important in the endemic situation. For example, age is the dominant heterogeneity in determining measles patterns in unvaccinated communities, but spatial and social factors are perhaps more important when infection is ephemeral. To prevent significant outbreaks, it is necessary to maintain a greater level of biological control, i.e., density-dependent factors, in the population than would have pertained had the infection been endemic. Thus, in rather simplified terms, immunization, which produces a functionally similar effect to infection, must maintain immunity levels above those at endemic equilibrium if epidemics are to be prevented and elimination maintained.

Eradication of Risk

Given that the aim is to eradicate, it would be irresponsible not to consider the consequences of eradication. After a period of time, the degree of susceptibility to infection builds up to levels which would result in a pandemic of infection should the pathogen return. For example, there are few, if any, individuals below the age of 15 years that have immunity to smallpox. Again, the most important measure is the degree of susceptibility in the host population as a measure of the current density dependence should the disease be reintroduced. The assessment of the risk is largely accomplished by assessment of the susceptibility of the population.

One of the perennial problems of public health is that when a risk of an epidemic has been correctly identified and successfully reduced, there is no way of telling if it was as a result of these efforts that nothing happened. This is an inconvenience in terms of public perception, but more of a problem in terms of modeling. If models are to be validated and used with confidence, in terms of assessing risk, then ideally, from a theoretical perspective, these risks should be measured without intervention. This paradoxical situation is likely to become increasingly important. Essentially, the reduction in infectious disease reduces the amount of data available to fit and validate models.

CONCLUSIONS

Mathematical models currently have a limited role in the process leading towards eradication of infectious diseases but a central role in the processes involved in the control of infectious diseases, which is a prerequisite to eradication. This role is largely through the interpretation of biological processes into epidemiological processes, and its relation to economic and social processes. Models can provide the link between immune responses and time horizons and discounting. The types of models required close to eradication are different from those required to design control programs and have received relatively little attention, particularly in relation to assessment of risk and consequences of outbreaks or changes in social factors.

Similar to the problems close to eradication are those of emerging infections, with the added complication that little is usually known about emerging infections. What is clear, however, is that eradication is best achieved prior to, or soon after, emergence. Perhaps more research effort is required to ascertain the risks of (potentially) emerging infections in order to aid eradication.

ACKNOWLEDGMENTS

G.F. Medley and D.J. Nokes are Royal Society University Research Fellows. W.J. Edmunds is a Wellcome Trust Training Fellow.

REFERENCES

Anderson, R.M., and R.M. May. 1984. Spatial heterogeneity and the design of immunisation programs. *Math. Biosci.* **72**:83–111.

Anderson, R.M., and R.M. May. 1991. Infectious Diseases of Humans. Oxford: Oxford Univ. Press.

Dushoff, J. 1996. Incorporating immunological ideas in epidemiological models. *J. Theor. Biol.* **180**:181–187.

Edmunds, W.J., C.J. O'Callaghan, and D.J. Nokes. 1997. Who mixes with whom? A method to determine the contact patterns of adults that may lead to the spread of airborne infections. *Proc. Roy. Soc. Lond. B* **264**:949–957.

Edmunds, W.J., G.F. Medley, and C.J. O'Callaghan. 1997. Social networks and the probability of catching a cold. *JAMA*, in press.

Edmunds, W.J., G.F. Medley, and D.J. Nokes. 1996a. Cost-effectiveness of hepatitis B immunisation (letter). *JAMA* **275**:907.

Edmunds, W.J., G.F. Medley, and D.J. Nokes. 1996b. The transmission dynamics and control of hepatitis B virus in a developing country. *Stat. Med.* **15**:2215–2233.

Edmunds, W.J., G.F. Medley, and D.J. Nokes. 1996c. Vaccination against hepatitus B virus in highly endemic areas: Waning vaccine induced immunity and the need for booster doses. *Trans. Roy. Soc. Trop. Med. Hyg.* **90**:436–440.

Gay, N.J. 1996. Analysis of serological surveys using mixture models: Application to a survey of parvovirus B 19. *Stat. Med.* **15**:1567–1573.

Guyatt, H.L., M.S. Chan, G.F. Medley, and D.A.P. Bundy. 1995. Control *of Ascaris* infection by chemotherapy: Which is the most cost-effective option? *Trans. Roy. Soc. Trop. Med. Hyg.* **89**:16–20.

Habbema, J.D.F., G.J. van Oortmarssen, and A.P. Plaisier. 1996. The ONCHOSIM model and its use in decision support for river blindness control. In: Models for Infectious Human Diseases: Their Structure and Relation to Data, ed. V.S. Isham and G.F. Medley, pp. 360–380. Cambridge: Cambridge Univ. Press.

Keeling, M.J., and B.T. Grenfell. 1997. Disease extinction and community size: Modeling the persistence of measles. *Science* **275**:65–67.

Margolis, H.S., P.J. Coleman, R.E. Brown, E.E. Mast, S.H. Sheingold, and J.A. Arevalo. 1995. Prevention of hepatitis-B virus transmission by immunisation: An economic analysis of current recommendations. *JAMA* **274**:1201–1208.

McLean, A.R. 1995. Vaccination, evolution and changes in the efficacy of vaccines — A theoretical framework. *Proc. Roy. Soc. Lond. B* **261**:389–393.

Medley, G.F. 1996. Conflicts between individual and communities in treatment and control. In: Models for Infectious Human Diseases: Their Structure and Relation to Data, ed. V.S. Isham and G.F. Medley, pp. 331–343. Cambridge: Cambridge Univ. Press.

Nokes, D.J., and R.M. Anderson. 1991. Vaccine safety versus vaccine efficacy in mass immunisation programmes. *Lancet* **338**:1309–1012.

Nokes, D.J., and J. Swinton. 1997. Vaccination in pulses: A strategy for global eradication of measles and polio? *Trends Microbiol.* **5**:14–19.

Williams, J.R., D.J. Nokes, G.F. Medley, and R.M. Anderson. 1996. The transmission dynamics of hepatitis-B in the UK: A mathematical model for evaluating costs and effectiveness of immunisation programmes. *Epidemiol. Infec.* **116**: 71–89.

Standing, left to right:
Karl-Otto Habermehl, Lex Muller, Graham Medley, Meinrad Koch, Frank Fenner, Jacob John
Seated, left to right:
Heinz Zeichhardt, Walter Dowdle, Steve Ostroff, Eric Otteson

5

Group Report: How Is Eradication to Be Defined and What Are the Biological Criteria?

E.A. OTTESEN, Rapporteur

W.R. DOWDLE, F. FENNER, K.-O. HABERMEHL,
T.J. JOHN, M.A. KOCH, G.F. MEDLEY,
A.S. MULLER, S.M. OSTROFF, H. ZEICHHARDT

INTRODUCTION

There are many issues related to eradication on which consensus has not been reached, but all agree on the need for clear, unambiguous definitions of terms. Without consensus on the meaning of eradication, elimination, control, and related terms, discussions will remain ambiguous and confused.

Similarly, the basic biological and epidemiological features of infectious agents that make them susceptible to eradication must be defined. With the eradication of smallpox, the uncertainty of whether infectious diseases *can* be eradicated has been replaced by the determination to target the infectious scourges of humankind that *are* eradicable. The challenge has been to identify the basic biological and epidemiological features that increase the likelihood of organisms being appropriate targets for eradication. Empiric experience with successful eradication efforts is limited to just one example, though ongoing efforts to eradicate Guinea worm and polio are providing many additional, useful lessons. Indeed, it is becoming clear that eradicability is not restricted to just one type of infectious agent or just one type of intervention tool. Thus, it is important to attempt to identify those biological or epidemiological features of diverse infectious agents that allow them to be considered as targets for eradication.

The Eradication of Infectious Diseases
Edited by W.R. Dowdle and D.R. Hopkins © 1998 John Wiley & Sons Ltd.

DEFINITIONS

Introduction

Public health efforts directed at infectious diseases can have different goals and achieve different levels of success. Indeed, there appears to be a distinct hierarchy in terms of our degree of mastery over infections, and it is these levels of mastery that are defined below. The important differences among them involve the distinction between disease caused by the infection and the infection itself, the level of reduction achieved for infection and/or disease, the need for long-term continuation of control efforts, and finally, the importance of the geographic area in defining the outcome of intervention efforts. What is specifically not addressed in these definitions is the relative desirability or feasibility of achieving different levels of disease reductions, nor the time required for establishing them.

Terms Defined

Control: Reduction of disease incidence, prevalence, morbidity or mortality to a locally acceptable level as a result of deliberate efforts; continued intervention measures are required to maintain the reduction.

Elimination of disease: Reduction to zero of the incidence of a specified disease in a defined geographic area as a result of deliberate efforts; continued intervention measures are required.

Elimination of infection: Reduction to zero of the incidence of infection caused by a specific agent in a defined geographic area as a result of deliberate efforts; continued measures to prevent reestablishment of transmission are required.

Eradication: Permanent reduction to zero of the worldwide incidence of infection caused by a specific agent as a result of deliberate efforts; intervention measures are no longer needed.

Extinction: The specific infectious agent no longer exists in nature or the laboratory.

Examples

Control: Diarrheal diseases and acute respiratory infections (in particular pneumonia and bronchiolitis) are life-threatening conditions, especially during childhood. Systematic control of mortality associated with these diseases may be achieved through the use of oral rehydration salts for diarrhea and antibiotics for pneumonia. Increasing attention is being paid to control of the incidence of diarrhea and pneumonia through new vaccines against rotavirus and bacterial agents as well as against *Haemophilus influenza* and pneumococcus, respectively.

Elimination of Disease: Infection with *Clostridium tetani,* a sporulating bacterium, is the cause of neonatal tetanus (NNT). The disease is due to a toxin secreted by the bacterium which resides and multiplies in the intestines of animals such as cattle and horses and is discharged into the environment by defecation. Bacterial spores survive and disseminate in soil and dust. Neonates are vulnerable to infection when, during an "unclean delivery," infection may be introduced by unhygienic conditions during preparation of the umbilical cord or from exposure to dust. Two broad interventions can prevent NNT: (a) aseptic care of the cord to prevent infection; (b) immunization of pregnant women with tetanus toxoid to ensure passive transfer of antitoxin antibodies to the neonates, preventing NNT even if they become infected. By applying both interventions for all deliveries, NNT *as a disease* can be eliminated. However, the infectious agent will continue to remain in the environment and can cause disease if protective measures are discontinued.

Elimination of Infection: In 1985 the Pan American Health Organization (PAHO) launched a program to eliminate polio from the Western Hemisphere. The last cases of indigenous polio had been recorded in the United States and Canada in 1979, but polio was widespread in many other countries of the Americas. The elimination strategy consisted of the following: (a) maintaining high levels of routine vaccination of children; (b) establishing National Immunization Days, carried out four weeks apart in the historically "low season" for polio, for all children five years of age regardless of vaccine history; (c) continuous clinical and laboratory surveillance to detect wild poliovirus infections; and (d) "mop-up" vaccination activities in high-risk areas where poliovirus was found to persist. The last case of paralytic poliomyelitis caused by the wild virus in the Americas was diagnosed in August, 1991. Polio was declared to be "eradicated" from the Western Hemisphere in 1994. Poliovirus continues to circulate elsewhere in the world and frequent reintroductions into the Western Hemisphere can be expected. Maintenance of the region as polio-free requires continuous high-level vaccine coverage and continuous surveillance for poliovirus.

Eradication: Smallpox was recognized as a severe human disease for many centuries. In 1958, the World Health Assembly (WHA) resolved to eradicate smallpox by vaccinating at least 80% of the population. This strategy succeeded in eliminating the disease from a number of previously endemic countries, but in 1966 there were still about 20 million cases and 1.5–2 million deaths per year. WHA then decided to launch an intensified smallpox eradication program with emphasis on surveillance and containment, the provision of adequate quantities of high-quality vaccine, and continued routine vaccination. In December, 1979, just over two years after the last known case of naturally acquired smallpox had been detected in Somalia in October, 1977, the Global Commission for Certification of Smallpox Eradication declared the world free of smallpox. The findings of the Commission were endorsed by WHA in May, 1980. Apart from two cases of smallpox occurring in August–September, 1978, in association with the use of smallpox virus in a laboratory in England, there has not been a case of smallpox in the world since then. Smallpox is the only disease to have been eradicated.

Extinction: There is as yet no example of the deliberate extinction of the causative agent of a human disease. Stocks of smallpox virus are held in high-security laboratories in the United States and Russia. In 1996 the WHA recommended that they be destroyed in June, 1999. If the recommendation is carried out, barring possible unknown sources, the virus will be extinct.

INDICATORS FOR POTENTIAL ERADICABILITY RELATED TO THE BIOLOGICAL AND EPIDEMIOLOGICAL ATTRIBUTES OF INFECTIOUS AGENTS

Introduction

The following discussion focuses on criteria important for *eradication*, although they may also relate to elimination or control; it focuses on the *infectious agents* themselves (and the tools necessary to approach them), not on the diseases they cause; finally, it focuses on *infections in humans*, even though many of the same principles related to human pathogens will apply to pathogens of animals as well.

In theory, if the "right tools" were available, all infections should be eradicable, but in reality, of course, there are distinct biological features of the organisms and technical factors in dealing with them that make their potential eradicability more or less likely; what is needed now is to identify these features.

Many biological attributes of infectious organisms relate to their potential eradicability, but these are often so intertwined and mutually dependent that *no single biological attribute* can be considered to be an "absolute" determinant of, or barrier to, potential eradicability; i.e., no single biological feature has been identified that would guarantee success or failure of eradication efforts. The reason, quite simply, is that even very formidable obstacles to eradicability (e.g., the existence of an animal reservoir) might be overcome completely if appropriate means were available (e.g., by eliminating the infection in that reservoir, as has been the case for rabies in Great Britain).

Similarly, it is obvious but still worthy of emphasis that today's categorization of diseases as potentially eradicable or not eradicable can change completely tomorrow, either because research efforts are successful in developing new effective intervention tools or because those presumed obstructions to eradicability that seemed so important in theory proved capable of being overcome in practice.

The Principal Indicators of Eradicability

Three indicators are considered to be of primary importance in determining the potential eradicability of infectious diseases; these are that:

- Effective intervention is available to interrupt transmission of the agent.
- Practical diagnostic tools with sufficient sensitivity and specificity are available to detect levels of infection that can lead to transmission.

- Humans are essential for the life cycle of the agent; the agent has no other vertebrate reservoir, and it does not amplify in the environment.

The first two indicators are essential elements for eradication of infection; the third is the biological property most often affecting potential eradicability of the organism.

Effective Intervention Tool

The effectiveness of an intervention tool has both biological and operational dimensions. Vaccines, therapeutic agents, behavioral modification, vector control, or a combination of these must be of sufficient efficacy to interrupt transmission of the agent and of sufficient global applicability to achieve eradication. Smallpox vaccine was an ideal intervention tool: effective, inexpensive, relatively stable, and easily administered by nonprofessional health personnel. Oral polio vaccine has many of the same qualities.

The conception of those qualities that constitute an effective intervention tool may change as more is learned about the biology and epidemiology of an agent and opportunities available for intervention. Polio and measles were once considered noneradicable; potential eradicability was demonstrated for both by innovative immunization strategies and subsequent national and regional elimination of indigenous infections.

Elimination validates the effectiveness of an intervention tool, but it does not necessarily make the agent a candidate for *eradication*. Transmission of *Treponema pallidum* has been eliminated in several developed countries by active syphilis surveillance and prompt treatment of infections. Other countries are likely to follow, but this strategy is an unlikely tool for global intervention at the present stage of health systems development in most areas of the world.

Diagnostic Tools

This element too has both biological and operational dimensions. The tools must be of sufficient sensitivity and specificity to detect infection that can lead to transmission and of sufficient simplicity to be applied globally by laboratories with widely ranging capabilities and resources. One of the initial attractions of smallpox as a target for eradication was that clinical presentations were almost pathognomonic, and no diagnostic laboratory tests were required. However, for the final stages of eradication and for eventual certification, specific laboratory diagnostic tests to distinguish varicella zoster from smallpox were critically important.

Conceptions of what constitutes an adequate diagnostic tool will also change as newer methods are developed and more is learned about the biology of an agent. For many years no reliable tools were available to distinguish vaccine strains from wild strains of poliovirus, a situation precluding eradication. Modern molecular technology now allows poliovirus isolates to be readily differentiated and to be further characterized as to genotype. This latter has important implications for implementing appropriate immunization strategies, and the potential barrier of test complexity is overcome by a hierarchical network of laboratories capable of performing tests at increasing levels of test specificity as needed.

Humans Are Essential for the Life Cycle

Eradication is most feasible as a target of deliberate intervention when humans form an essential component of the agent's life cycle, because it is then possible to apply an effective intervention tool to humans and disrupt transmission and agent multiplication. To date, the most successful eradication campaigns have been directed against pathogens such as smallpox, poliomyelitis, and Guinea worm whose only vertebrate reservoir is humans. By contrast, despite the availability of an excellent vaccine for yellow fever effective in eliminating urban infection, the existence of a nonhuman primate host has prohibited eradication of the infection.

While agents which have a life cycle independent of humans or which have the capacity to multiply independently outside of humans (e.g., yellow fever, cholera, *C. tetani*) are much more difficult eradication targets, even these attributes are relative and not absolute barriers to eradication. It is necessary only that the independent reservoir can also be targeted with an effective intervention tool, as in the examples of successful regional elimination for some pathogens (i.e., rabies elimination from Great Britain and *Schistosoma japonicum* elimination in Japan), or of diseases in which the alternative animal reservoir is a domestic species where infection can often be eliminated regionally by a combination of veterinary and medical public health measures. Indeed, possibilities for such elimination are enhanced by simplicity of the extra-human cycle (e.g., only one host) and low transmission potential.

Biological/Epidemiological Considerations Related to Potential Eradicability

In addition to the three principal indicators of eradicability, a number of other criteria affect the feasibility of eradication. Since infectious diseases are geographically heterogeneous, elimination will be easier in some localities than in others, and the criteria listed below relate to the ease with which elimination would be possible. In some circumstances these properties may make local elimination (and therefore eradication) impossible, but they are different from the principal indicators in that they may determine local, rather than global, barriers to elimination/eradication (see Hinman and Hopkins, this volume, for additional details).

Transmission Potential

Infectious agents are transmitted from individual to individual; those that are not easily transmitted are more easily eliminated. The most useful measure of transmission is the *basic reproduction number* (R_0), defined as the number of secondary cases from one infectious case in a completely susceptible population; a component of this quantity for vector-borne infections is the *vectorial capacity*. The basic reproduction number is inversely related to the proportion of the population that remains unexposed, i.e., the higher the value, the lower the average age of infection and the smaller the proportion unexposed.

R_0 has essentially three components determining its value: the duration of infectiousness of an individual, the rate of "contacts" made between individuals within a population, and the probability of infection when a contact occurs. For vector-borne infections the number of contacts is determined by the density of appropriate vectors, and for sexually transmitted infections by the rate of sexual partner acquisition. Consequently the value of R_0 is determined by the environment/behavior of a particular population; there is no "absolute value" for R_0.

This quantity does, however, reflect the "effort" that must be put into eradication. For example, for directly transmitted viral infections, the critical proportion of the population that must be immunized to achieve herd immunity is $(1-1/R_0)$. In localities or populations where R_0 is small, a lower vaccination proportion is required for elimination than in other localities where transmission rates are extremely high. Thus, for example, measles transmission rates are high in densely populated regions with high birth rates, and consequently immunization coverage will have to be close to 100% to achieve elimination. Indeed, in a particular locality, the current intervention tools might not be adequate, and additional measures may be required to reduce the transmission rate to enable elimination. Thus, the effectiveness of intervention tools (the first principal indicator) should be measured in relation to the transmission potential, and different strategies may be required in different areas.

Susceptibility to Reinfection

Where elimination (and eradication) success depends on the ability to create sufficient levels of immunity within a population to block transmission (especially through immunization), the potential to develop solid, sterile "natural" immunity is beneficial. If an agent is unable to infect the same individual twice (e.g., smallpox), immunization can be targeted at those individuals yet to be infected (essentially children). Where natural immunity is unable to prevent reinfection (e.g., gonorrhea) the whole population (exposed and unexposed) must be targeted. Generally, agents which do not induce solid acquired immunity have a higher prevalence of infection (e.g., helminth infection vs. virus infections). Intermediate between these extremes may be those infections that induce transient immunity or decreased infectiousness on reinfection (e.g., rotavirus, RSV). The development of vaccines for such infections will likely be more difficult as they will have to be more effective than natural immunity; consequently, eradication efforts will have to focus more heavily on chemotherapy and/or behavior change and/or environmental modification (e.g., helminth infections, and the current Guinea worm eradication program).

Proportion of Infections That Are Clinically Detectable

The presence of clinical manifestations in a high proportion of those infected will enhance the potential for eradication for two distinct reasons. First, high case morbidity/mortality rates will increase the perceived burden of the disease and positively impact on the political and social will to achieve eradication. Second, it relieves some of the diagnostic burden from supporting laboratory services.

Amplification in a Vector

While amplification in a vector generally increases a pathogen's transmission potential, the presence of a vector may also represent a target for environmental change to reduce transmission potential. Indeed, because reduction of vector density decreases transmission both to and from the vector, it has a multiplicative effect on reducing the transmission potential; for example, halving the vector density will reduce the transmission potential to one-quarter of its original level.

Duration of Infectiousness and Recrudescence

If the intervention method is primarily based on prevention of transmission by induction of immunity (i.e., vaccination) or by environmental/behavioral change rather than by cure of infection (e.g., through chemotherapy), then the primary duration of any elimination program increases with the duration of infectiousness. For example, hepatitis B virus (HBV) with infectiousness lasting many decades in the carrier state will require many decades to be eliminated from any population while those infected (and infectious) cannot be cured. Likewise, the existence of recrudescence of infectiousness (e.g., *varicella zoster* virus [VZV]) represents a similarly (though discontinuous) long infectious period. The eradication of smallpox took approximately 100 infectious periods. A similar requirement would represent a programmatic barrier to the eradication of HBV, VZV, and tuberculosis, among others.

As the duration of a program increases, its likelihood of success decreases for economic, societal, and political reasons. A long time scale also generates biological reasons for reduced success, including the increased chance of development of "resistance" and escape mutants to vaccine-induced immunity. On the other hand, a long infectious period can also provide a potential target for very effective intervention. For example, the development of chemotherapy or therapeutic vaccines to cure, reduce, or prevent infectiousness of HBV or VZV would greatly reduce the required vaccination coverage and the necessary time scale of any program. However, effective use of such interventions requires that diagnostic tools are available to detect infection throughout the full infectious period (including any "quiescent" periods), as they are for HBV, but not VZV. It may be possible that such chemotherapy interventions alone are sufficient tools for eradication, as in the case of certain helminth infections. In these situations, the life expectancy of the parasite can be considered approximately equivalent to the duration of infectiousness, so that *Schistosoma spp.* (life expectancy thought to be about five years) are likely more easily eradicated, than *Ascaris lumbricoides* (about one year), since the target intervention period is longer for *Schistosoma* and the chemotherapy need not be repeated so frequently to derive the same chance of killing each adult parasite.

Geographic/Ecologic Restriction

Smaller geographic distribution and greater ecologic restrictions imply greater feasibility for both elimination and eradication. Indeed, eradication proceeds by successive geographic elimination, thereby continually reducing the scale of the problem.

Environmental Persistence

Environmental persistence of pathogens is conceptually equivalent, in terms of affecting feasibility of eradication, to the duration of infectiousness (see section above on *Duration of Infectiousness and Recrudescence*); increasing survival of infectious stages generally increases the required duration of any eradication program. (Note that significant *multiplication* of the organism in the environment without appropriate control tools precludes eradication.)

Seasonality/Epidemic Periodicity in Incidence

Seasonality is the annual cycling of incidence due to environmental (including climatic) changes. The precise role of seasonality in development of programs is dependent on the characteristics of agent and intervention method, but its existence has been exploited successfully in both the smallpox and polio eradication programs.

Epidemic periodicity is caused by infection dynamics and again may be exploitable. However, successful intervention programs will alter the "natural" periodic pattern.

Long-term Effectiveness of Interventions

As infectious agents are subject to evolutionary adaptation, and any intervention imposes a selective advantage on variants capable of circumventing that intervention, the potential to develop "resistance" will always be an important consideration. Experience shows that such development is especially likely for chemotherapeutics and insecticides, so that eradication programs based on one such agent alone are likely not to be successful. Consideration needs to be given to how multiple drugs (or insecticides) should be applied; in parallel, in series or with a combination of methods.

The generation of escape mutants able to overcome vaccine-induced immunity appears to be a potential problem in those agents displaying antigenic variation and may constitute a barrier to eradication (e.g., with HBV). Genetic variability may also decrease the effectiveness of diagnostic tools.

Relatedness of Other Agents

The relatedness of the target organism to other species may also be an important consideration affecting eradicability. While there is a continuum from agents having no known "nonhuman" relatives (such as polio and mumps viruses), other organisms (such as *A. lumbricoides*) have relatives which may pose diagnostic problems or even be involved in infection and transmission between humans. Given, especially, the diagnostic problems posed by these latter organisms, it may be inappropriate to consider them as potentially eradicable.

Genetic Reversion of Live Virus Vaccines

The probability of genetic reversion of attenuation to pathogenicity must always be considered in the application of live vaccines. Measles vaccine virus appears to be highly stable based on the experience of many years of use. Genetically less stable are polio vaccine viruses with evidence of reversion following long-term shedding in immunocompromised vaccinees or multiple passages in nonimmune populations. Reversion has little programmatic consequence in highly immunized populations, but must be carefully weighed in devising strategies for cessation of immunization.

Niches and Natural Ecosystems

Species in any natural ecosystem are interdependent, and each species may be said to occupy an ecological niche. If such niches are determined by interactions with other species as well as by environmental considerations, then removal of one species might affect the balance among remaining species. It is sometimes argued that each infectious agent occupies an ecological niche and that removal of a species from that niche will inevitably result in adaptive changes in other species, either currently prevalent or newly emerging, to fill that niche; i.e., eradication is pointless since new infections will arise. The argument can be refuted on several grounds.

Most importantly, there is no good empirical evidence that such niches are important for different pathogenic species *on a relevant time scale*. Smallpox was successfully eradicated twenty years ago, polioviruses have been eliminated from the Americas for several years, and rabies from the U.K. for approximately 100 years. No species have yet filled those potential niches. Furthermore, the emergence of new infections, such as human immunodeficiency virus, suggests that niches may remain unfilled for very long periods due to the adaptive barriers to development of a significant transmission potential within host populations.

Certainly, it is possible that many species, and strains within species, are competitive, such that reduction in the incidence of one pathogen results in the increased incidence of an antigenically related pathogen. Some evidence suggests such a relationship between yaws and syphilis, and it is possible that the eradication of smallpox led to human monkeypox infections, although it is much more likely that humans have always been accidental hosts for monkeypox which was unrecognized against a background of smallpox. Nonetheless, in most cases the pathogens benefiting from this "competitive release" will be less well adapted and thus easier to control (and eradicate) than those primarily targeted. Furthermore, the precise interaction between species can only be demonstrated by disturbance of the equilibrium; curtailing eradication programs because other pathogens *might* increase in incidence is not scientifically or ethically tenable.

Laboratory Containment of Eradicated Agents

The definition of eradication implies that the etiologic agent is no longer a threat to humans. For Guinea worm disease, eradication is virtually synonymous with extinction since the agent cannot replicate outside its human host. For smallpox virus, poliovirus, measles virus, and those agents which may be replicated *in vitro*, eradication in the absence of extinction requires sufficiently stringent laboratory containment policies and facilities to prevent deliberate or accidental human infection and subsequent reintroduction of the disease. Maintenance of a vaccine stockpile provides additional assurance of disease containment in the event of deliberate or accidental infection.

The Listing of Infections as Potentially Eradicable or Noneradicable

Examples of infectious agents that can be considered potentially eradicable in accord with the principal indicators discussed above include those listed in the Recommendations of the International Task Force for Disease Eradication (CDC 1993) as the causative agents of dracunculiasis, poliomyelitis, lymphatic filariasis, mumps, rubella, and taeniasis/cysticercosis. Certainly, this is not a final or comprehensive list. To the contrary, classification of an agent as eradicable or noneradicable is a dynamic, evolving process. Agents classified as noneradicable based on current knowledge, technology, and health systems development may be reclassified as conditions change. Shortcomings in one of the three principal elements of eradicability may be overcome by the strength of one or both of the remaining two. Poliomyelitis was once considered noneradicable because of the large number of clinically inapparent infections. This factor became less crucial after introduction of laboratory-based surveillance of acute flaccid paralysis and the successful demonstration that "pulse" mass immunization interrupted transmission.

At the time the 1993 Recommendations were prepared, measles was listed as noneradicable. Three years later measles was eliminated from South America and is now considered by many international health authorities as a promising candidate for eradication following polio. Hepatitis B has also been proposed as a strong candidate for eradication, requiring universal immunization and time. And there will be others.

Because any ranking or listing of agents as eradicable or noneradicable is time limited, we have resisted the temptation to create still another list. We predict that the top candidates for eradication in the future, as in the past, will be self-selecting as the three principal elements are met. Selection of a candidate agent as a target for eradication and the development of the necessary global commitment are complex social and political processes, as discussed in the other three group reports (see Hall et al., Cochi et al., and Goodman et al., this volume).

DISCUSSION

Five levels of our "mastery" over infectious agents have been defined. Distinguishing between eradication and extinction as separate entities has been an attempt to divorce public health issues from ecological and ethical discussions over maintenance of biodiversity. The principal argument for avoiding extinction of any species is that it stands for the deliberate destruction of biodiversity which is against the central tenet of current global, ecological consensus (the Rio de Janeiro Agreement). The distinction between elimination of infection and elimination of disease has the obvious implication that the former is more difficult to achieve than the latter. Any outcome of deliberate public health efforts not definable as either elimination or eradication is recognized as having achieved a particular level of "control." Another term in common parlance, "elimination of (the disease) as a public health problem," is one that refers to situations with a level of disease control that is very high. No attempt was made in our deliberations to define this term formally, and its use is not felt to be necessary to the development of eradication targets, strategies, or programs.

The search for indicators related to the biological or epidemiological features of infectious agents that could identify the potential eradicability or noneradicability of organisms has led to a conclusion that the biological property most often affecting potential eradicability of the organism is the agent's essential dependence on humans for its life cycle (i.e., there being no other vertebrate reservoir and its not amplifying independently in the environment). Overriding this biological determinant, however, are the absolute requirements for an effective intervention agent and for tools to diagnose the infection sufficiently to detect any incidence of infection. These three criteria can be applied to candidate organisms to identify those that may be considered as potentially eradicable, but it was recognized that the experience with successful eradication is so limited that theoretical predictions might well be wrong and that probably the best predictor of eradicability is the demonstration of feasibility in eliminating infection from a specified region. Thus, any list of organisms considered potentially eradicable or noneradicable (e.g., that generated by the International Task Force for Disease Eradication [CDC 1993]) should be considered only as a guideline for focusing on those factors either favoring or limiting potential eradication of the infectious agent.

Experience has also taught that "potential eradicability" or "noneradicability" are concepts that are ever evolving and are not labels that can be applied with certainty to any infectious agent (except smallpox). Polio, measles, and hepatitis A are all infections now considered to be potentially eradicable, whereas just a few years ago the tools or understanding necessary to make such projections were not available. What is most clear, now, is that there is a definite need for periodic reassessment of different organisms for their potential eradicability and, indeed, a clear imperative to focus our research on objectives that would overcome those factors that presently appear as barriers to eradication.

REFERENCE

CDC (Centers for Disease Control and Prevention). 1993. Recommendations of the International Task Force for Disease Eradication. *Morbid. Mortal. Wkly. Rep.* **42 (RR–16)**:1–38.

6

Disease Eradication Initiatives and General Health Services: Ensuring Common Principles Lead to Mutual Benefits

R.B. AYLWARD[1], J.-M. OLIVÉ[1], H.F. HULL[1],
C.A. DE QUADROS[2], and B. MELGAARD[1]

[1]Global Programme for Vaccines and Immunization, World Health Organization,
20 Avenue Appia, 1211 Geneva 27, Switzerland
[2] Special Program on Vaccines and Immunization, Pan American Health Organization,
525 23rd Street NW, Washington, D.C., U.S.A.

ABSTRACT

The most frequently cited criticism of disease eradication initiatives is that they hamper the establishment and strengthening of other health services by diverting scarce human and financial resources. This chapter reviews the eradication efforts that have been conducted against yellow fever, yaws, malaria, smallpox, dracunculiasis, and poliomyelitis to determine whether such initiatives invariably compromise health systems in general.

Overall, the legacy of eradication initiatives suggests that they provide excellent opportunities to strengthen national health infrastructures. On occasion, however, these opportunities may have been squandered in the haste to eliminate the target disease. With each new eradication effort there appears to be increasing attention to the impact on other health programs as well as a growing awareness of the need to exploit these initiatives to benefit health systems in general.

Since their inception, eradication initiatives have been inextricably tied to the development of primary health care (PHC) in developing countries. Early initiatives, such as those directed against yellow fever and malaria, focused international attention on the lack of access to basic health services. Either by design or default, all eradication initiatives, particularly the ongoing program to eradicate poliomyelitis, have supported the five PHC principles: equitable distribution, community involvement, focus on prevention, appropriate technology, and a multisectoral approach. There remains, however, a lack of studies which objectively evaluate the impacts of these initiatives on other health programs, especially in terms of the allocation of resources.

The Eradication of Infectious Diseases
Edited by W.R. Dowdle and D.R. Hopkins © 1998 John Wiley & Sons Ltd.

INTRODUCTION

The most frequently cited criticism of disease eradication initiatives is that they hamper the establishment and strengthening of other health services (CDC 1993). Such initiatives, the argument runs, divert meager human and financial resources from public health programs and primary health care (PHC) (Yekutiel 1981). In complete opposition to this criticism is the position of disease eradication advocates who state that "strengthening the public health structure of the world" is a primary reason for undertaking these efforts (Foege 1984).

In this chapter we undertake to evaluate whether disease eradication initiatives are inherently good or bad in terms of their impact on health systems in general. We have attempted to determine whether recent or ongoing initiatives reflect the lessons that have been learned from previous eradication efforts. We review the effect of the six major disease eradication initiatives of this century on other health services (Table 6.1), with particular attention given to developing countries.

DISEASE ERADICATION INITIATIVES AND THE
DEVELOPMENT OF HEALTH SERVICES

The implementation of eradication initiatives and the development of health services have often been closely intertwined, particularly in developing countries (Soper 1965; Meheus and Antal 1992). Beginning with the attempt to eradicate yellow fever from the Western Hemisphere in the early 1900s, the greatest common obstacle for such initiatives has been the lack of a strong health infrastructure worldwide (Soper 1965; Farid 1980; Fenner et al. 1988). Subsequently, most eradication initiatives have invested considerable resources to strengthen the limited health care systems that do exist, often resulting in sustained improvements (Farid 1980; Fenner et al. 1988). In Central Africa, for example, the yaws control and eradication programs of the 1950s have been seen as "... the starting point for the system of basic health services" (Meheus and Antal 1992).

In the haste to establish the health services needed to eliminate a specific disease, however, early eradication initiatives have in some countries devoted enormous funds to the training and hiring of "uni-purpose" health workers. The malaria eradication initiative of the 1950s and 1960s, in particular, is frequently cited as having developed a whole cadre of workers whose sole purpose was to implement the strategies needed to conduct surveillance for, and eliminate, the *anopheles* mosquito (Gish 1992). Although the malaria eradication program resulted in huge reductions in the leading cause of morbidity and mortality of many countries, upon the cessation of this ultimately unsuccessful initiative, many of those workers were ill-suited, and not motivated, to undertake more general health work. The initiatives that followed the malaria eradication program, however, have had a much different legacy with respect to their impact on health personnel.

Table 6.1 Major eradication initiatives launched against human diseases in the 20th century and examples of their impact on health services.

Eradication Initiative	Years*	Certification of Eradication	Examples of the Impact of the Eradication Initiative on Other Health Services
Yellow fever (*Aedes aegypti*)	1915–1977	No	Developed the first nationwide administrative health systems in many countries. Established first international committment to solving a common health problem. Eliminated the malaria vector *Anopheles gambiae* from Western Hemisphere and Egypt.
Yaws	1954–1967	No	Acted as the foundation for the delivery of basic health services in many unserved areas. Improved national surveillance for other diseases of public health importance. Demonstrated other health activities could be combined with eradication programs.
Malaria	1955–1969	No	Led to 1978 world summit on PHC by exposing poor state of basic health services. Established and/or strengthened the health infrastructure in many countries. Routinely solicited support for health programs from the highest political levels.
Smallpox	1958–1980	Yes	Established a model for the planning and implementation of public health programs. Served as the basis for establishing the global Expanded Programme on Immunization. Trained an international cadre of health workers in epidemiology and surveillance.
Dracunculiasis	1986–ongoing	—	Facilitated the delivery of basic health services in unserved areas and areas of conflict. Formalized ongoing community involvement in health activities in underserved villages. Provided clean water, health education and health workers/volunteers in unserved areas.
Poliomyelitis	1985–1944 1988–ongoing	Americas —	Established the strategies and political will to undertake global eradication of polio. Developed ICC mechanism to improve the mobilization and allocation of resources. Exploited and strengthened the multisectoral approach to solving of health problems. Established global laboratory network which can be used for other health initiatives.

* Except for the yellow fever initiative and the polio initiative in the Americas, this refers to the years of the global eradication programs. National and/or regional initiatives always preceded the global efforts.

PHC = primary health care; ICC = Interagency Coordinating Committees

Although the successful smallpox eradication program of the 1960s and 1970s depended on a huge number of persons who were trained specifically to undertake that program, upon cessation of the initiative many went on to senior health management positions in their countries (Fenner et al. 1988). Of the remaining "ex-smallpox" workers, a substantial number joined the newly launched Expanded Programme on Immunization and are credited with it "now standing ... as one of the great health achievements of this century" (Henderson 1994). The ongoing polio eradication initiative relies almost exclusively on existing surveillance, immunization, and laboratory personnel, providing them with extensive training in general disease control skills, as well as the strategies needed to eradicate polio (Birmingham et al. 1997). A basic principle of the dracunculiasis eradication initiative is the establishment of at least rudimentary PHC in underserved areas (CDC 1994; Hopkins and Ruiz-Tiben 1991).

Even the unsuccessful malaria eradication initiative may have ultimately had a substantial positive impact on the development of health services in that it highlighted "the sad and skeletal rural health structure of developing countries" (Farid 1980). This focusing of international attention on the need to strengthen PHC systems worldwide (Warren 1990; Gish 1992) contributed directly to the universal endorsement of the PHC concept at Alma-Ata in 1978 (WHO 1978).

PROMOTING THE PRINCIPLES OF PRIMARY HEALTH CARE THROUGH DISEASE ERADICATION INITIATIVES

The 1978 Alma-Ata Conference codified the five basic principles of PHC as equitable distribution, community involvement, focus on prevention, appropriate technology, and a multisectoral approach (Warren 1990; WHO 1978). Most of these same principles have been promoted by the major disease eradication initiatives, particularly the more recent smallpox, dracunculiasis, and polio efforts (Table 6.2).

Eradication initiatives promote the concept of equity in health care by potentially freeing all persons in perpetuity from risk of the target disease. These efforts usually mandate the delivery of health services to the world's most underserved populations as eradication requires that at least surveillance for the target disease reaches virtually every population subgroup in the world (CDC 1994; Hopkins 1985). Eradication initiatives demonstrate the importance and feasibility of delivering health services to populations that are living in areas often considered too remote or too sparsely populated to warrant the investment that would be needed to establish and maintain routine health services. It has even been suggested that eradication initiatives, such as those targeting yaws and dracunculiasis, promote equity in health services delivery by using the presence of the disease in a community as an indicator of inadequate PHC (Foege 1984; Kumar 1982). Eradication initiatives also promote equity in health care delivery through the ceasefires which have been negotiated to reach civilian popula-

Table 6.2   Relationship between eradication initiatives, the basic principles of primary health care, and the infrastructure needed for the delivery of health services.

Basic Principles of Primary Health Care*	Relative Importance to Eradication Initiatives**	Components of Health Services Infrastructures	Relative Importance to Eradication Initiatives**
Equitable distribution	++++	Information systems	++++
Community involvement	++++	Management	++++
Focus on prevention	++++	Manpower development	+++
Appropriate technology	+++	Logistics	++++
Multisectoral approach	+++	Health facilities	+
		Research	+++

*   Sources: WHO (1978); Warren (1990); Smith and Bryant (1988)
** On a relative scale of + (less important) to ++++ (most important).

tions that have been isolated by fighting in countries such as the Sudan, El Salvador, and Afghanistan (CDC 1995; Day 1996; Hull 1997).

Community involvement has been an essential feature of all of the eradication initiatives undertaken to date, although the nature of that involvement has depended on the complexity of the particular eradication strategy. In many countries, community leaders, members, and volunteers have been primarily responsible for the successful implementation of eradication strategies, ranging from disease surveillance in the smallpox eradication program (Fenner et al. 1988), to health education during the dracunculiasis eradication effort (CDC 1994) and vaccine delivery during the National Immunization Days (NIDs) for polio eradication (Hull et al. 1994). An evaluation of the Americas polio eradication program ranked social mobilization, including community organization and leaders' involvement, as the area where the impact on other health programs was greatest (Taylor Commission 1995).

It has been suggested that the "community mobilization," which was part of these initiatives, may on occasion have amounted to "community manipulation" in that the community was only involved in implementing the strategies. However, a basic tenet of a disease's "eradicability" is that it is perceived as a serious health problem in both donor and endemic countries (CDC 1993). In addition, the ongoing eradication initiatives targeting dracunculiasis and polio, as well as the smallpox program, provide ample examples of how the strategies have been adapted to address other health priorities in individual countries or communities (Figure 6.1). For example, NIDs for polio eradication have been exploited to deliver not only oral polio vaccine, but interventions ranging from iodized salt in Iran to anti-helminthics in Mexico. The delivery of clean water and other basic services is a key element of the dracunculiasis eradication program.

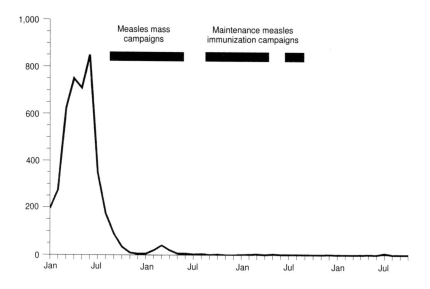

Figure 6.1   One outcome of the smallpox eradication program was the interruption of measles transmission in the Gambia, demonstrating the potential to eliminate another leading cause of childhood mortality. Source: Foster and Pifer (1971).

Eradication programs inherently promote the concept of disease prevention as their ultimate purpose is the "reduction of the worldwide incidence of a disease to zero" (CDC 1993). In addition to raising awareness of disease prevention among the general population, eradication initiatives also promote the concept among policy and decision makers (Fenner et al. 1988; Gish 1992). With the recognition that support from the highest political levels is essential to the success of an eradication initiative (Yekutiel 1981), advocacy efforts targeting those levels are now a basic component of eradication strategies (Fenner et al. 1988; Hull et al. 1994).

Among the criteria used to determine the eradicability of a disease is the existence of appropriate technology in the form of a practical intervention that is "effective, safe, inexpensive, long-lasting, and easily deployed" (CDC 1993). Whether ultimately successful or not, all of the eradication initiatives have shown the potential to achieve substantial reductions in illness and disease through the use of relatively simple technologies (Yekutiel 1981). During the smallpox eradication program, simple devices such as disease recognition cards demonstrated how complex health concepts could be brought to illiterate populations through the use of appropriate technologies (Fenner et al. 1988).

Disease eradication initiatives also demonstrate both the importance and feasibility of securing multisectoral support for health programs. In particular, the nationwide immunization campaigns of both the smallpox and polio eradication initiatives required collaboration that went far beyond the health sector to Ministries such as defense, planning, transport, and education, to find the personnel, vehicles, fuel and other equipment, and expertise needed to coordinate such massive events (Fenner et al. 1988; de Quadros 1994). Eradication initiatives have also provided an opportunity to promote the participation of the private sector in health programs (Olivé et al. 1997). In the Philippines, for example, the polio eradication initiative received tremendous support from over 150 private corporations which provided personnel, facilities, transport and other resources for the NIDs (Tangermann et al. 1997).

STRENGTHENING HEALTH SERVICES THROUGH DISEASE ERADICATION INITIATIVES

The delivery of all health services requires a "functional infrastructure" comprised of information systems, management, manpower development, logistics, facilities, and research (Smith and Bryant 1988). Although the relative importance of individual components might differ, the same basic infrastructure is required for the implementation of any disease eradication initiative (Table 6.2). Overall, the relationship between eradication initiatives and other health services seems to have been a symbiotic rather than parasitic one in that the resources and attention that eradication initiatives have invested in this infrastructure have benefited many aspects of health services in general (Figure 6.2).

Information systems are the most important component of any disease eradication

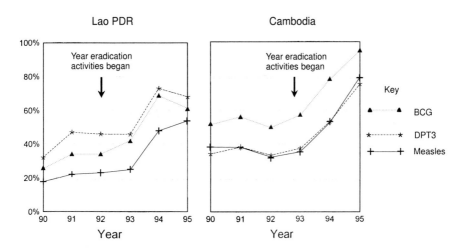

Figure 6.2 In countries of the Western Pacific routine infant immunization coverage has risen significantly since the implementation of polio eradication activities (Aylward et al. 1997). [Note: The Kingdom of Cambodia and the People's Democratic Republic of Lao were the only countries of the Western Pacific which had routine immunization coverage of less than 50% and conducted polio eradication activities.]

initiative, and usually the most difficult to establish. Timely surveillance must be combined with ongoing program monitoring to target future activities accurately and respond to the changing epidemiology of the disease (Fenner et al. 1988). The same capacity to gather and analyze information is critical to the success of PHC and public health programs in general (Smith and Bryant 1988). Eradication initiatives train public health and PHC staff in the basic concepts of disease reporting, case investigation, laboratory investigation, case follow-up, and information management (Fenner et al. 1988). As noted previously, the epidemiological skills learned by eradication workers can only be transferred to other disease control priorities if adequate attention is given to ensuring the broader perspective of such staff (Ladnyi et al. 1983; Litsios 1993).

Because disease eradication initiatives require the rapid development of accurate and timely information systems, it has sometimes been necessary to establish, at least temporarily, autonomous surveillance systems. Although it has been suggested that this leads to a duplication of effort within Ministries of Health, or worse, compromising the original health information system, this perspective seldom reflects the reality of the circumstances in which eradication initiatives work or their long-term intentions. During the yellow fever eradication initiative, a specific surveillance system was developed due to the lack of any other information system at that time in the targeted countries (Soper 1965). Similarly, although national disease surveillance existed in many of the countries which implemented drancunculiasis eradication activities, the affected villages were often outside the formal health sector (Hopkins and Ruiz-Tiben 1991). More recently, the polio eradication initiative has needed to temporarily establish parallel information systems in some developing countries because of the low value placed on timely surveillance data (Nareth et al. 1997). The intention and practice has been to use these systems as a basis for either establishing or strengthening national information systems.

From as early as the 1950s, the program to eradicate yaws was conducted in conjunction with surveillance for diseases such as leprosy, African sleeping sickness, onchocerciasis, and dracunculiasis (Hopkins 1985). More recently, the polio eradication initiative has demonstrated the capacity for health services in general to benefit from information systems that were established to facilitate an eradication effort. In Cambodia, a nationwide, geographically representative, timely reporting system for polio began detecting measles outbreaks even prior to the planned expansion of the system to include other diseases of public health importance (Nareth et al. 1997). During the 1991 cholera epidemic in Peru, health authorities took advantage of the surveillance system that had been established to support polio eradication to facilitate the immediate, nationwide reporting of suspected cholera cases (de Quadros 1994).

The development of management capacity and systems has invariably been regarded as one of the major strengths of disease eradication programs (Yekutiel 1981; Soper 1965; Farid 1980; Fenner et al. 1988; Taylor Commission 1995). Just as invariable has been the use of those same management skills to facilitate the delivery of other health services. In 1930, the Yellow Fever Service in Brazil was successfully directed against the recently introduced malaria vector, *Anopheles gambiae*, in large part because "it was the only organized administrative health service in the region at the time capable of taking action against this new threat" (Soper 1965). The principles of program management employed in the smallpox eradication program continue to be a model for the implementation of health programs worldwide (Fenner et al. 1988). In the Americas, the only formal study that has evaluated the impact of an eradication initiative on health systems in general stated that the management strategies of the polio eradication initiative "worked and contributed to other programs, either sharing them or setting the example and becoming a model to learn from" (Taylor Commission 1995). Immunization authorities in the countries of the Americas region now "present yearly and five-yearly national plans of action which outline objectives, activities, and expected results, with identification of both costs and funding sources" (de Quadros 1994).

Disease eradication initiatives can play a particularly valuable role in facilitating the development of health manpower for the most underserved areas of a country as well as at more central levels. This investment in human resources is probably best seen in the yaws and dracunculiasis programs, where the diseases are virtually limited to rural, underserved, and often sparsely populated regions (Meheus and Antal 1992; CDC 1994; Hopkins and Ruiz-Tiben 1991). Due to the nature of the diseases and the eradication strategies, both initiatives required the training of local personnel for the implementation and long-term follow-up of the program (Hopkins 1985; Kumar 1982). In addition to providing the first regular contact with health services in some areas of Asia and Africa, these "eradication" personnel have worked with local populations on health education, clean water supplies, and other PHC fundamentals (Hopkins and Ruiz-Tiben 1991).

One of the principal obstacles to the routine delivery of basic health services in many countries is the logistics of ensuring an ongoing supply of the appropriate equipment to the appropriate place at the appropriate time. Eradication initiatives can substantially contribute to overcoming these obstacles for a number of reasons. First, as noted above, eradication initiatives teach the management skills required to plan, budget, and identify properly those resources needed for implementing a health program (Farid 1980; Fenner et al. 1988). Second, as special programs, eradication initiatives are able to bring substantial new resources to logistical problems, in the form of vehicles, computers, communications materials, cold chain, and other equipment, all of which can also be used for the delivery of other PHC materials (Soper 1965; Farid 1980; Fenner et al. 1988). Third, eradication initiatives demonstrate the role other sectors can play in solving logistical difficulties (Fenner et al. 1988; Hull et al. 1994).

Ongoing research has played a fundamental role in all eradication initiatives. Development of the viscerotome during the yellow fever eradication effort allowed the systematic investigation of all persons who died of fever (Soper 1965) while the introduction of the bifurcated needle substantially simplified the work of the intensified smallpox eradication program after 1968 (Fenner et al. 1988). In addition to establishing new technologies, eradication programs have also contributed to the development and dissemination of epidemiological tools; the "cluster sampling" method, which is now widely used for estimating immunization coverage and other health indicators, was operationalized during the smallpox program (Henderson et al. 1973). As well as demonstrating the relevance of research to public health programs, eradication initiatives teach basic research principles and skills to health personnel through epidemiological studies and the evaluation of new technologies (Fenner et al. 1988; Litsios 1993).

The impact of eradication initiatives on some aspects of a health infrastructure can be readily measured in terms of the number of information systems established or the manpower trained. Many impacts cannot be readily quantified, however, but have an even greater effect on child survival and the delivery of health services in the long term. The success of eradication initiatives increases the prestige of the health sector, raises the motivation of health workers, and establishes the political will to tackle other major health problems (Fenner et al. 1988; Taylor Commission 1995). Following the eradication of polio in the Americas, for example, the Ministers of Health launched an initiative to eradicate measles, one of the leading causes of preventable childhood mortality, from the Western Hemisphere by the year 2000 (de Quadros et al. 1996).

IMPACT OF ERADICATION INITIATIVES ON RESOURCE AVAILABILITY FOR OTHER HEALTH SERVICES

Despite the substantial overlap in the guiding principles and necessary infrastructure for both eradication initiatives and health services delivery in general, many persons voice a concern that eradication programs compromise the strengthening of health systems by diverting scarce human and financial resources (CDC 1993; Yekutiel 1981).

Eradication initiatives require a tremendous investment in human resources to establish the management capacity and information systems needed to implement the strategies (Soper 1965; Farid 1980; Yekutiel 1981; Fenner et al. 1988; Hopkins and Ruiz-Tiben 1991). As discussed earlier in this chapter, the recruitment and training of personnel specifically for eradication programs has left a varied legacy in that some of these workers were subsequently ill-suited for more general health work. This was primarily a feature of the earliest initiatives, however, as more recently eradication workers have routinely been absorbed into the existing health structure or used as a basis for establishing services in areas where none previously existed (Farid 1980; Fenner et al. 1988; Ladnyi et al. 1983; Hopkins and Ruiz-Tiben 1991). Because of the development of national health infrastructures, it has been possible to implement the most recent eradication initiative, targeting poliomyelitis, primarily through existing health staff (de Quadros 1994). Although this has sometimes caused the temporary diversion of personnel from their primary responsibilities during activities such as

NIDs, the gains in experience and motivation have usually offset this brief interruption in routine activities (Taylor Commission 1995).

Although eradication initiatives require the investment of substantial financial resources in the short term, the long-term savings due to the cessation of control activities and decreased burden of the target disease has the potential to release substantial sums for the improved delivery of other health services (Ladnyi et al. 1983; Bart et al. 1996). Virtually any disease eradication initiative will eventually prove cost effective as the savings continue to accrue in perpetuity (CDC 1993). In addition, much of the "eradication funds" are actually spent on transport and cold chain equipment and the strengthening of logistics, information systems, and other components of the health services infrastructure.

Some of the early eradication initiatives, particularly those targeting yellow fever and malaria, undoubtedly caused the reallocation of a substantial proportion of the budgets of national governments, international organizations, and donor agencies from other health priorities (Farid 1980; Gish 1992). Unfortunately, there is a dearth of hard data to document either the extent of such reallocations or the impact they had on overall morbidity and mortality. For both historical and ongoing eradication initiatives, it is especially difficult to determine what proportion of the national or international resources allocated to these programs would otherwise have been available to the health sector.

Each eradication initiative has spent a substantial proportion of its time and effort seeking new funding sources (Soper 1965; Fenner et al. 1988). The more recent initiatives have been particularly innovative in this regard and have also established novel mechanisms to ensure the most efficient use of available donor support (de Quadros 1994). The polio eradication initiative has received substantial assistance from Rotary International, an international service club organization, which developed a "PolioPlus Programme" to help the initiative through advocacy, vaccine purchase, cold chain support, and social mobilization (Hull et al. 1994). In 1985, major donor agencies with an interest in polio eradication in the Americas joined with national governments in establishing Interagency Coordinating Committees (ICCs) to ensure the coordination of activities (Figure 6.3) (de Quadros 1994). ICCs have now been established in all World Health Organization regions and in some countries have begun to consider other aspects of maternal and child care. As noted in the example of the Philippines, the polio eradication initiative has also sought and received substantial resources from the private sector (Tangermann et al. 1997).

In the Americas up to 80% of the costs of polio eradication are covered by national resources (de Quadros 1994), while in poorer countries, particularly in Africa, more than 50% of the overall requirement comes from external sources. In all countries, however, these national resources represent in large part opportunity costs in the form of regular staff salaries, facility maintenance, and transport. Of the national resources used to cover actual financial costs, the majority would probably not be available for other health programs due to the diversity of the funding sources and their motivations for providing assistance. National funds for such things as fuel, training of volunteers,

R.B. Aylward et al.

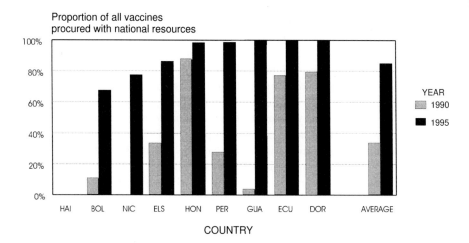

Figure 6.3 Since the institution of Interagency Coordinating Committees (ICCs) and National Plans of Action with the polio eradication initiative in the Americas, there has been a substantial increase in the proportion of all childhood vaccines procured with national resources. Countries that were not self-sufficient in procurement prior to 1990: Haiti (HAI), Bolivia (BOL), Nicaragua (NIC), El Salvador (ELS), Honduras (HON), Peru (PER), Guatamala (GUA), Ecuador (ECU), Dominican Republic (DOR).

and social mobilization originate not from a single central source but from a myriad of national, state, district, and village sources in both the public and private sectors. Although it is relatively easy to raise multisectoral support from all levels for time-limited mass campaigns which offer nationwide visibility, it is much more difficult to secure such assistance for ongoing routine health programs (Yekutiel 1981).

CONCLUSIONS

The majority of the literature on the impact of eradication initiatives on general health services is anecdotal, hypothetical, or speculative. While some eradication initiatives, particularly those conducted before the mid-1970s, may have diverted both human and financial resources, there is little documentation. Most importantly, the impact of such effects on overall morbidity and mortality in the targeted countries is not known. Additional efforts are needed to quantify objectively the impacts of eradication initiatives on other health programs, especially in terms of the allocation of resources.

The evidence which does exist, however, suggests that the disease eradication initiatives which have been undertaken since the turn of the 20th century have played a major role in focusing international attention on the need to strengthen health services in general. In addition to supporting the basic principles of primary health care, these initiatives have often contributed directly to the strengthening of health infrastructures, especially in the poorest countries. The provision of essential services will continue to be the focus of international health efforts (Bobadilla and Cowley 1995), but ethical, technical, political and, increasingly, economic arguments will ensure the adoption of new disease eradication goals. The challenge ahead is to ensure that the principles which are common to disease eradication initiatives and basic health services culminate in mutual benefits.

REFERENCES

Aylward, R.B., J. Bilous, and R.H. Tangermann, et al. 1997. Strengthening routine immunization services in the Western Pacific through the eradication of poliomyelitis. *J. Infec. Dis.* **175 (Suppl. 1)**:S268–S271.

Bart, K.J., J. Foulds, and P. Patriarca. 1996. Global eradication of poliomyelitis: Benefit-cost analysis. *Bull. WHO* **74(1)**:35–45.

Birmingham, M.E., R.W. Linkins, B.P. Hull, and H.F. Hull. 1997. Poliomyelitis surveillance: The compass for eradication. *J. Infec. Dis.* **175 (Suppl 1.)**:S146–S150.

Bobadilla, J.L., and P. Cowley. 1995. Designing and implementing packages of essential health services. *J. Intl. Dev.* **7(3)**:543–554.

CDC (Centers for Disease Control and Prevention). 1993. Recommendations of the International Task Force for Disease Eradication. *Morbid. Mortal. Wkly. Rep.* **42 (RR–16)**:1–38.

CDC. 1994. Update: Dracunculiasis eradication — Mali and Niger, 1993. *Morbid. Mortal. Wkly. Rep.* **43(4)**:69–71.

CDC. 1995. Implementation of health initiatives during a cease-fire: Sudan, 1995. *Morbid. Mortal. Wkly. Rep.* **44(23)**:433–436.

Day, M. 1996. Conflicts threaten polio target. *New Sci.* 11 May, p. 7.

de Quadros, C.A. 1994. Strategies for disease control/eradication in the Americas. In: Vaccination and World Health, ed. F.T. Cutts and P.G. Smith, pp. 17–34. Chicester: Wiley.

de Quadros, C.A., J.-M. Olivé, and B. Hersh, et al. 1996. Measles elimination in the Americas: Evolving strategies. *JAMA* **275**:224–229.

Farid, M.A. 1980. The malaria programme — From euphoria to anarchy. *World Hlth. For.* **I(1,2)**:8–33.

Fenner, F., D.A. Henderson, I. Arita, Z. Jezek, and I.D. Ladnyi. 1988. Smallpox and Its Eradication. Geneva: WHO.

Foege, W.H. 1984. Feasibility of eradicating yaws. *Rev. Infec. Dis.* **7(Suppl. 2)**:S335–S337.

Foster, S.O., and J.M. Pifer. 1971. Mass measles control in West and Central Africa. *Afr. J. Med. Sci.* **2**:151–158.

Gish, O. 1992. Malaria eradication and the selective approach to health care: Some lessons from Ethiopia. *Intl. J. Hlth. Serv.* **22(1)**:179–192.

Henderson, R.H. 1994. Vaccination: Successes and challenges. In: Vaccination and World Health, ed. F.T. Cutts and P.G. Smith, pp. 3–16. Chicester: Wiley.

Henderson, R.H., H. Davis, D.L. Eddins, and W.H. Foege. 1973. Assessment of vaccination coverage, vaccination scar rates, and smallpox scarring in five areas of West Africa. *Bull. WHO* **48**:183–194.

Hopkins, D.R. 1985. Control of yaws and other endemic treponematoses: Implementation of vertical and/or integrated programs. *Rev. Inf. Dis.* **7(Suppl. 2)**:S338–S342.

Hopkins, D.R., and E. Ruiz-Tiben. 1991. Strategies for dracunculiasis eradication. *Bull. WHO* **69(5)**:533–540.

Hull, H.F. 1997. Pax polio. *Science* **275(3)**:40–41.

Hull, H.F., N.A. Ward, B.P. Hull, J.B. Milstein, and C. de Quadros. 1994. Paralytic poliomyelitis: Seasoned strategies, disappearing disease. *Lancet* **343**:1331–1337.

Kumar, S. 1982. Guinea worm eradication programme and Primary Health Care. *J. Comm. Dis.* **14(3)**:212–215.

Ladnyi, I.D., Z. Jezek, and A. Gromyko. 1983. Five years of freedom from smallpox. *J. Hyg.* **27(1)**:1–12.

Litsios, S. 1993. Which way for malaria control and epidemiological services? *World Hlth. For.* **14**:43–51.

Meheus, A., and G.M. Antal. 1992. The endemic treponematoses: Not yet eradicated. *World Hlth. Stat. Qtly.* **45**:228–237.

Nareth, L., B. Aylward, O. Sopal, D. Bassett, M.C. Vun, and J. Bilous. 1997. Establishing AFP surveillance under difficult circumstances: Lessons learned in Cambodia. *J. Infec. Dis.* **175 (Suppl. 1)**:S173–S175.

Olivé, J.-M., J.B. Risi, and C.A. de Quadros. 1997. National Immunization Days: Experience in Latin America. *J. Infec. Dis.* **175 (Suppl. 1)**:S189–S193.

Smith, D.L., and J.H. Bryant. 1988. Building the infrastructure for primary health care: An overview of vertical and integrated approaches. *Soc. Sci. Med.* **26(9)**:909–917.

Soper, F.L. 1965. Rehabilitation of the eradication concept in prevention of communicable diseases. *Pub. Hlth. Rep.* **80(10)**:855–869.

Tangermann, R., M. Costales, and J. Flavier. 1997. Poliomyelitis eradication and its impact on Primary Health Care in the Philippines. *J. Infec. Dis.* **175 (Suppl. 1)**:S272–S276.

Taylor Commission. 1995. The impact of the Expanded Program on Immunization and the Polio Eradication Initiative on health systems in the Americas. Washington: Pan American Health Organization.

Warren, K.S. 1990. Tropical medicine or tropical health: The Heath Clark Lectures, 1988. *Rev. Infec. Dis.* **12(1)**:142–156.

WHO (World Health Organization). 1978. Report of the International Conference on Primary Health Care, Alma-Ata, U.S.S.R., September, 1978. Geneva: WHO.

Yekutiel, P. 1981. Lessons from the big eradication campaigns. *World Hlth. For.* **2(4)**:465–490.

7

Economic Appraisal of Eradication Programs: The Question of Infinite Benefits

A.K. ACHARYA and C.J.L. MURRAY

Harvard Center for Population and Development Studies,
9 Bow St., Cambridge, MA 02138, U.S.A.

ABSTRACT

Economic appraisal of disease eradication gives rise to the particular problem of making decisions between programs for which benefits accrue in perpetuity. If the benefit is assessed through methods other than monetary evaluation of life (e.g., through a quality of life year measure instead) and without the discounting of future benefits, we observe that it accrues to an infinite level. This chapter suggests solutions to this problem, and concludes that the present society should set aside funds which it then uses to undertake eradication programs. The eradication programs can be prioritized according to the burden from the relevant disease and the cost of controlling that disease.

INTRODUCTION

Economic appraisal of health interventions, whether delivering health services or health research activities, usually takes one of two forms: cost-effectiveness analysis or the closely related method, cost-benefit analysis. In this chapter, we will briefly outline the logic of these two methods and then explore the special problems that emerge when applying these tools to eradication programs. To foreshadow the main body of the chapter, special analytical problems exist when undertaking economic appraisal of health interventions because the benefits of an eradication program may at times be infinite. If the benefits are not infinite in nature, then the economic appraisal of eradication programs can proceed as it would for any other health intervention. If the benefits, however, are infinite, various options must be examined. The infinite stream aspect of benefits remains whether we see the eradication program globally, which this volume identifies as "eradication," or within a region or a nation, which is called "elimination" in this volume.

The Eradication of Infectious Diseases
Edited by W.R. Dowdle and D.R. Hopkins © 1998 John Wiley & Sons Ltd.

ECONOMIC APPRAISAL OF HEALTH INTERVENTIONS

In the field of health, the dominant mode of economic analysis of health interventions is cost-effectiveness analysis (World Bank 1993; Jamison et al. 1993; Gold et al. 1996). In cost-effectiveness analysis, the costs of an eradication program, such as polio immunization intervention measured in US dollars or in another currency unit, are compared with the benefits of an intervention measured in some general unit of health outcome or even control. Standard methods have been developed to define the costs of interventions based on the economic concept of opportunity cost. The opportunity cost of the resources used in an intervention is the value of the best foregone use of those resources. In other words, resources only have an opportunity cost in a world where wants exceed available resources. Most cost-effectiveness studies count all costs to society of an intervention and not simply the costs to the provider. Benefits of interventions can be measured using a wide variety of health outcomes such as deaths averted, potential years of life saved, quality-adjusted years of life (QALY) and most recently, disability-adjusted years of life (or DALY — a type of standardized QALY).

The results of a cost-effectiveness analysis are expressed as a cost-effectiveness ratio: usually dollars per QALY gained or dollars per DALY averted. Several broad reviews of cost effectiveness of different interventions have been undertaken in high-income (Tengs et al. 1994) and developing countries (Jamison et al. 1993). These studies show that the cost effectiveness of health interventions varies by many orders of magnitude. In an analysis of 500 life-saving interventions in the U.S.A., Tengs et al. (1994) found cost-effectiveness ratios varying from nearly 0$ per year of life saved to over 10 billion US$ per year of life saved. Likewise, Jamison et al. (1993) reported variation in cost-effectiveness ratios for 50 interventions of four to five orders of magnitude. The interpretation of the results of any given cost-effectiveness analysis including cost-effectiveness analysis of eradication programs depends on the threshold cost that society is willing to spend to save a year of life. In a low-income country, society may only be willing to pay a GDP (gross domestic product) per capita to save a year of life (as low as US$ 300 in some countries) while in richer countries society may be willing to spend several multiples of GDP per capita to save a year of life.

This threshold value often remains implicit in the policy debate on intervention choice; several methods have been used by economists, however, to try an define the monetary value of various types of health benefits. In cost-benefit analysis, the dollar value of various health benefits is estimated so that both the costs and benefits of a health intervention are calculated in dollars. In many areas of economic appraisal such as industrial investment and education, cost-benefit analysis is the standard method in use. In health, however, many decision makers and public health practitioners have been very reluctant to quantify health benefits in dollar terms. This reluctance to use cost-benefit analysis as opposed to cost-effectiveness analysis is probably based on more than simply a reluctance to attach a precise dollar value to years of healthy life but also based on some of the inequitable assumptions that lie at the heart of cost-benefit methods. Dollar valuations of health outcomes have been developed using primarily two conceptual approaches: the willingness-to-pay (WTP) approach and various human capital approaches.

The Willingness to Pay Approach

In the absence of markets for health states which could directly provide information on the "price" of health, economists have proposed methods for estimating the value that individuals attach to improvements in health or extensions in survival. Based on the principles of welfare economics, one can attempt to calculate the willingness to pay or accept compensation to achieve some decrease or increase in probability of losing one's life. Then, in evaluating value of a life year, a decision maker should take into account a person's willingness to pay for a year of life plus the net social contribution this individual makes to the society beyond the personal evaluation of her life. We first examine the methods proposed by economist to measure value of life and argue that this is an untenable method of evaluation in many situations.[1]

The fundamental premises of the WTP approach are based on the assumption that social welfare is based on individual welfare functions since social decisions should reflect the interests, preferences, and attitudes to risk of those who are likely to be affected by the decisions (Mishan 1982). Another feature of these studies is that they essentially measure the value of changes in the probability of death. The immediate task is to examine this last aspect of WTP approach; we will come back to the issue of what should be included in the accounting of social welfare. Since we are essentially concerned with government's role in elimination or eradication, the appropriate social welfare function should take into account the welfare or the WTP evaluations made by all people except those we find absolutely deplorable, for example, the person who would enjoy seeing the suffering and death of great many people.

In the WTP approach, it is usually meaningful to measure the willingness to forego some small reduction in probability of death by simply noting the marginal rate of substitution between wealth level and risk level. What is being valued is the change in risk of death based on *ex-ante* assessment of life. It has been shown that willingness to pay for reduction in risk of death is most likely to increase with wealth; safety is a normal good, i.e., people consume more of it as income rises.

None of these models seek to discover the willingness to pay for a year of life under certainty. In fact there is good reason to believe that this drawback makes WTP approach particularly unsuited for use in analysis of research toward disease eradication through vaccine or new drug development, especially if the case fatality rate is

---

1 This section received considerable input from a literature survey as a part of Kenji Shibuya's on-going dissertation project at the Harvard School of Public Health.

significantly high for the disease in question. This can be seen fairly clearly in a simple WTP model.

Consider health states that are very different from death, i.e., health states that are essentially good but can be ranked fairly clearly; for example, a not so unhealthy 30-year-old man who can achieve greater health if he eats more healthy expensive food along with joining the health club, etc. Then indexing most of his health status as fairly positive, the demand for health goods can be seen in the following way according to the following diagram:

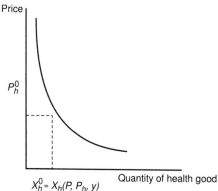

$X_h^0 = X_h(P, P_h, y)$ Quantity of health good

Figure 7.1 A demand curve for a health good.

where P_h denotes price of health, P is the vector of prices of all other goods, X_h is the demand for the health good which produces health through function f, and y is the income. The area left of the demand curve above the price is the consumer surplus. The value or the utility to the consumer of this purchase is the consumer surplus plus the rectangle formed by the origin, P_b^0, X_h^0 and the Cartesian coordinate (X_h^0, P_h^0). Notice that at an infinite price none of this good is purchased resulting in 0 value to the consumer.

For any change in price the consumer experiences a change in utility, both through a real change in income due to the price change and through the relative evaluation of all the different goods he/she consumes. The willingness to accept the old price can be seen by removing (for a price decline) or adding (for a price rise) an amount income that would keep this individual's utility at the old price. We can essentially write the compensation, CV, implicitly, in the following way, where x denotes vector of goods other than health goods, V denotes utility and is essentially a function of income and prices through purchasing of goods:

$$V(P, P_h^1, y - CV) = V(P, P_h^0, y) = V\left(x\left(P, P_h^0, y\right), f\left(X_h(P, P_h^0, y)\right)\right). \quad (7.1)$$

Even if price approaches infinity, note that CV is still defined since $V(x, f(0))$ is meaningful; i.e., $f(0) = 0$. In this case CV is meaningful for every possible vector of prices.

Now consider an essential drug or a vaccine in the absence of any curative care with near 100% case fatality rate. Let the price approach infinity, then the person dies and CV is not defined since V is now negative infinity. Hence, as soon as a person contracts this disease, the willingness to pay for recovery is undefined. The argument here is relevant as long as the case fatality is relatively high. Further, the point is not that V is negative infinity for a price approaching infinity, but that whenever the vaccine is not affordable, CV is not defined.

The WTP approach is essentially based on the idea that social decision should reflect the interests, preferences, and attitudes to risk of those who are likely to be affected by the decision. It is not clear from the outset who the affected parties are. And it is not clear that individuals view social projects solely from the viewpoint of private gains (for arguments regarding social and private discount rate, see Feldstein 1964; Marglin 1963; and Sen 1961).[2] Our result above shows that adding up individual CV's for cases where individuals face near certain death is meaningless.

The WTP analysis for risk reduction in death is essentially stated in the partial equilibrium form in that, say for vaccine development, it would simply add up individual CV to assess desirability of such research and development. It ignores economy wide impacts, such as the fact that prolongation of life is not costless to a society and affects intergenerational transfers. Arthur (1981) explores what would happen if such concerns were taken into account. He shows that welfare gains associated with a risk reduction in age-specific risks consists of three forces affecting consumption and some offsetting factors. The gains due to consumption due to lengthened life, increased productivity, and increased number of offspring is offset by the fact that increased consumption in later years must be financed by someone else's decreased consumption. In this sense one might argue then that willingness to pay is essentially the sum of all factors in a society that are affected by a disease.

An incorrect approach that may stem from Arthur's observation regarding the willingness to pay to recover from an illness is the cost of illness approach. This approach can be called the GDP opportunity cost, which we will next examine.

The Cost of Illness

The major alternative for monetizing the value of a year of life is often identified with studies of human capital. In these studies, the dollar value of a health gains is related to the costs of medical care averted and the discounted value of future earnings is embodied in various cost of illness studies (Rice 1994). In their original intent, the cost of illness approach to valuing health gains is based on the concept of GDP opportunity

---

2 A related point is made by Zeckhauser (1975): when decisions are made in public domain, the normative significance of what would be produced by a private market is diminished.

cost. Simply put, how much bigger would current and future GDP be if an intervention is applied or, in the case of cost of illness studies, if a disease were completely eliminated. As currently implemented, cost of illness methods deviate from strict GDP opportunity cost because of a number of aspects of the method that many users of the results have found objectionable.

Some analysts have suggested that the cost of illness serves as a lower bound of individual willingness to pay (Conley 1976). Presumably, an individual's willingness to pay to avoid a health risk includes at least foregone earnings due to illness plus the medical expenditures that would be averted. Individual willingness to pay will also include an extra component, quite likely to be large, such that the individual is willing to pay for the health gains per se. Thus, individuals with no future earnings, such as retired individuals, will nevertheless pay substantial sums to extend life or improve the quality of life.

While calculations of the present value of average future foregone earnings can be undertaken easily, whether these calculations even adequately capture the GDP opportunity cost is in doubt. The existence of unemployment entails, from a societal point of view, that most afflicted workers are replaceable. A worker currently unemployed can always gain employment due to the death or disability of the afflicted worker to obtain a net change in social earning of zero. Hence, the GDP opportunity cost of losing individuals may be close to zero or simply the transfer payment made to the disabled and/or their dependents. Further, if we allow for labor mobilization across borders, the productivity level of very few workers will be indispensable.

For developing countries where communicable diseases afflict mostly the unskilled workers and the unemployed, which number greatly, the cost of illness of a major cause of death and disability may be small. Bloom and Mahal (1997) report that the loss to GDP due to the widespread AIDS epidemic in many African nations is not detectable.

Since the question here concerns the role of government in conducting eradication programs, if a correct social WTP amount for a life can be worked out, then it would be easy to conclude when such efforts are desirable or more desirable than some other action for some other disease or for some other life saving intervention. It could be that a correct willingness to pay would be derived very differently from the one that takes into account only the private benefits. A social willingness to pay would be derived from the individual views of what it means to be a member of a society. Though it would evaluate death negatively, each death will be treated anonymously; hence, the social counterpart of V in Equation 7.1, when one is unable to afford treatment, would not be negative infinity. In fact, the concept of statistical life would be appropriate for social evaluation, yet deriving social values in this instance is impossible in practice.

ISSUES UNIQUE TO THE EVALUATION
OF ERADICATION PROGRAMS

The most widely accepted method of economic appraisal in the health sector is cost-effectiveness analysis. For the remainder of this chapter, we will explore the unique analytical challenges that emerge in cost-effectiveness studies of eradication programs. The basic problem is simple: the benefits of an eradication program may be infinite and, if they are infinite, the cost-effectiveness ratio for such programs will be near zero regardless of the cost in the numerator. Compared to other interventions that have finite costs and benefits, and thus nonzero cost-effectiveness ratios, eradication programs will appear much more attractive. All health resources available to society should in such a scenario be devoted to efforts that may lead to disease eradication — a permanent sustained reduction in the burden of a given disease. Such efforts would, therefore, include eradication programs and more generally some health research efforts. The unappealing conclusions that all health resources should be diverted from curative and preventive interventions to fund research and eradication programs follows immediately from infinite benefit streams. The critical analytical question to address is whether, from today's perspective, the benefits of an eradication program are indeed infinite. A second question is: if they are infinite, is there some way to avoid concluding that all health resources should be devoted to these efforts? Third, how do we choose a course of actions when nearly all actions yield infinite benefits?

Our exploration of the infinite benefits problem will proceed along the following lines. First, we may be able to conclude that no stream of benefits from eradication is truly infinite because of secular trends or risks of extinction. Even if benefits may in fact be infinite in selected cases (e.g., the economic practice of discounting future benefits), the present value of this infinite stream may transform into a finite quantity. This prompts the well-debated question as to whether or not health benefits should be discounted and if so on what grounds. If indeed the benefit stream is infinite, how then should we choose actions that affect infinite streams? If the infinite streams dominate all current care, what is then the legitimate level of sacrifice that the current generation should be willing to make to improve health conditions for all future generations? Finally, if society sets aside a sum of money that is dedicated to improve the health of future generations through eradication programs and health research, how do we choose between different eradication and research efforts — all of which may have infinite benefits?

Are the Benefits of Disease Eradication Infinite?

In most cases, there are two reasons why infinite benefit streams are not likely to arise. First, the incidence and mortality of many, if not most, diseases are decreasing due to socioeconomic development. The exact causal pathway by which socioeconomic changes lead to reductions in the incidence, case-fatality rates, and mortality rates from many infectious diseases and a number of noncommunicable diseases is not always known but the historical record of the last half century is clear. If socioeconomic development is expected to continue, and incidence and mortality from a disease is expected to decline progressively, then the benefits of eradicating this disease are finite. Programs that eradicate such diseases can be evaluated using the standard methods of cost effectiveness. It still may be the case, if the secular trend is slow, that the benefits of eradication are very large and would justify very large investments in eradication using standard cost-effectiveness criteria. In most regions of the world, trends for communicable, maternal, perinatal, and nutritional deficiencies are quite strongly declining so that eradication programs for most of these conditions will not have infinite benefit streams.

Even if the incidence and mortality from a condition is expected to remain constant, there is a small but real uncertainty about the survival of society. Asteroids may hit the earth, and in the long run we know that the sun and the solar system have a finite lifespan. In fact, because of this unavoidable uncertainty of the existence of society and even the earth, no stream of health benefits from eradication is truly infinite. Nevertheless, the stream of benefits from eradication may be very large and the cost-effectiveness ratios of devoting huge sums to eradication of health research may be so close to zero that conclusions similar to infinite benefit streams will be reached. The "discount rate" implied by the uncertainty of the survival of society is a very small number so that the area under an exponential decay with such a discount rate may be large compared to the annual size of the burden of disease. We must conclude that in no case will the benefits of an intervention, whether eradication or health research, be infinite. The rest of this discussion turns on the situations where the benefits of eradication are nevertheless very large.

Discounting Future Health Benefits

It is currently standard practice in cost-effectiveness analyses of health interventions to discount future health benefits (Gold et al. 1996; Jamison et al. 1993). Discounting is the practice whereby a year of life or a QALY or DALY in the future is discounted compared to a QALY or DALY today. The usual form of discounting is an exponential decay of the form: where t indicates time, r is the exponential rate of discount. As time increases, this values tends to zero no matter what the DALY value at some later time is. The area under this curve is finite even as time increases limitlessly:

$$\int_0^\infty e^{-rt}(DALYs_t)dt < \infty.$$

The rates most often used in cost-effectiveness analyses are 3–5%. In such cases, an infinite stream of one year of life saved every year would have a present value equal to 20 to 33 years of life. The effects of discounting at rates as high as 3 or 5% are, therefore, dramatic. Two programs of equal cost — one that eradicates a disease and one that simply cures a disease for one year — will differ in cost-effectiveness ratios by only one to two orders of magnitude using the discount rates commonly in use.

The rationale for discounting health benefits has been the focus of considerable controversy (Keeler and Cretin 1983; Lipscomb 1989; Redelmeier and Heller 1993; Weinstein and Stason 1977). Two arguments in favor of discounting have received the most attention (Lipscomb et. al. 1996): the time paradox and the consistency argument. Both of these arguments in favor of discounting future health benefits are consequentialist arguments. They do not claim that future health benefits are inherently less important, only that the consequences of not discounting future health states while discounting future costs are either counter-intuitive or inconsistent. We will briefly review these two arguments and, based on a more extensive analysis reported elsewhere, conclude that they are not very convincing.

The time paradox proposed by Keeler and Cretin (1983) is essentially the argument that postponement of expenditure on health would entail a higher number of saved lives in the future years due to interest earned on the saved expenditure. If society values health the same way every period, then postponement of expenditure would entail improved cost efficiency as expenditure on health is pushed forward indefinitely into the future. They show that since cost borne in present value terms on a project is always less when postponed one year hence and the health benefit is the same when postponed and not discounted, it always pays to defer a health intervention program. One would thus never implement a health intervention program. The paradox disappears only if cost of health and benefit are discounted at the same rate.

Weinstein and Stason (1977) offer an argument based on consistency for discounting future life years in cost-effectiveness analysis:

> [Since health states] are being valued relative to dollars and, since a dollar in the future is discounted relative to a present dollar, so must a life year in the future be discounted relative to a present dollar . . . . It is the discounting of dollar costs, and the assumed steady-state relation between and the assumed steady-state relation between dollars and health benefits, that mandates the discounting of health as well as dollars. (p. 720)

Under this view, future health states should be discounted exponentially at the rate of interest in the economy just as future cost is assessed in its present value.

Both of these justifications for discounting depend on highly restrictive and implausible assumptions about the degrees of freedom faced by decision makers. For example, in the time paradox argument, we are asked to imagine that intervention opportunities last for ever, and that allocation of health budget is at the policymaker's disposal for all time. In the case of the consistency argument, it seems that the health policymaker is also making the decision as to the optimal level of investment in capital for the entire economy, since he must take into account the rate of return on investment. (see Acharya and Murray 1997). At best, discounting future health benefits can be challenged and at worst, discounting health benefits should be rejected.

Near-Infinite Benefits Revisited

If the benefits of eradication are near-infinite or are simply extremely large and discounting at high rates as the normal practice in cost effectiveness is not justified, we are left with the unacceptable conclusion that all or nearly all of society's health resources should be devoted to research and eradication programs. Such a conclusion calls upon the current generations to make an excessive sacrifice of their own health for the health of future generations. While some degree of sacrifice between generations is reasonable, there is clearly some point at which sacrifice by one group for another can be deemed to be excessive (Parfit 1984). If one were behind a veil of ignorance, not knowing the generation to which you belonged, and you were asked about the legitimate level of sacrifice that a given generation should make for the health of future generations, you would clearly not choose to spend all health resources on the good of future generations. Following Rawls' (1971) you might choose to maximize the well-being of the generation that is likely to be worst off. If there are secular trends towards improved health, such a view might lead you to set aside only a small fraction of resources for the health of future generations because they are likely to be better off anyway.

The theoretical and practical solution to this problem of excessive sacrifice would be to set aside a fixed share of health resources devoted to improving the health of future generations through research and eradication efforts. In fact, most societies behave as if they have such a fixed share of health resources set aside for research activities. Investments in eradication efforts, on the other hand, have often come from budgets for current health intervention rather than such set-aside funds as for research. Based on dollars for research, the fraction of health resources set aside for improving the health of future generations is rather low — globally only a few percent of health resources are for research and development. The low fraction set aside by society overall may be due to several factors: the high discount rate of politicians largely concerned with outcomes prior to the next election, the moral urgency of addressing the problems of society now as compared to problems of society in the future, who are expected to be better off, or simply the selfishness of current generations.

Even if there are set-aside funds, how does one prioritize between various research and eradication efforts that may all have very large benefits? Cost-effectiveness ratios for various research and eradication options may all be extremely close to zero. Further, how do we exactly define legitimate sacrifice?

From the economic literature on the optimal savings rate for society, there are analytical methods that have been used to deal with infinite or near-infinite benefits which also say something concerning legitimate sacrifice. These methods are worth examining briefly as possible methods to deal with near-infinite benefit streams. Suppose that a society is concerned with intergenerational well-being and values the welfare of each generations equally — in other words society does not have a positive rate of pure time preference, it does not discount future utility. If the returns to investment remain positive, society will be led to conclude that little or no resources should be spent on current consumption and nearly all resources should be invested to increase the size of output in the future and thus consumption of future generations. Short of insisting on discounting future utility, several authors, including Ramsey (1928), have proposed methods to avoid the conclusion that the current generation should be required to undertake excessive sacrifice.

One way to get around this problem is to assume that if expenditure on consumption approaches zero at any period, then the society's utility in that period is negative infinity. Further, this requires an additional assumption that the society no longer simply maximizes well-being but the deviation from a targeted minimum. These two provisions are due to Koopmans (1965), who modified Ramsey's idea that the society should minimize deviation of consumption from a bliss point, the point where increase in consumption yields no further value to the society. These two provisions allow positive expenditure on consumption in all periods without discounting future utility and they should not be considered entirely implausible. It seems reasonable that a society would require some minimal expenditure to survive, and if a society is extinct then in the subsequent periods utility in actuality will have to be zero, though this latter fact does not follow from the mathematical formulation of the problem.

Koopmans' condition entails that the society should undertake positive expenditure to carry out interventions in the current period as well as setting aside expenditure on research for disease eradication. For if it did not, then it can improve the stream of welfare simply by making sure that health expenditure for every period is positive. Further, the society cannot gain further benefits beyond a certain point if it accumulated all its health resources which are completely left unused.

Another way of getting around the problem of near-infinite benefits is to adopt the view that policymaker will only be concerned with a finite time horizon, say, from current time to some time in the future called T. It may seem here that we have ended up discounting all periods after T at an infinite rate. It is not so because we can allow the policymaker to deal with future concerns by specifying what economists might call the salvage value of the policy. That is, we must specify an arbitrary terminal condition so that the policy instrument would leave the economy with specified productive resources. A condition by which the policymaker is constrained in his/her resource allocation problem is that the policy be designed so that at the end of the planning period, the economy is left with a certain specified amount of resources at its disposal.

Under this scheme applied to the analysis of an eradication, benefits accruing before T will be given equal weights to the benefits accruing from all types of current medical care. However, some resources, say, an amount equaling the average resource every year prior to T, will have to be in tact for the generations beyond T. The infinite stream of benefit due to disease eradication does not have to be explicitly taken into account. Subsequent planning interval periods follows T.

To summarize, we are left with three distinct arguments: benefits are not infinite, benefits are likely to be infinite but we can adopt a particular type of legitimate sacrifice argument which ensures that current health conditions are treated, and finally, the shortening of the planning period. Another approach is simply that every generation set aside funds for eradication and choose programs within that fund. This would entail that we choose a course of action from a set of actions which yield infinite benefits. This is possible through the use of von Weizsäcker (1965) overtaking criterion. Use of this criteria, however, does not always yield an answer. If we take the idea of setting aside funds for eradication program seriously and the overtaking criterion does not always yield an answer, can we still find a way of characterizing how one should go about pursuing eradication policy? The answer is yes. We turn to that answer next.

HOW TO CHOOSE BETWEEN ERADICATION PROGRAMS

We emphasize that because eradication programs may provide externalities across borders, the focus here is on eradication, not elimination. The eradication program is to be funded from a set-aside fund, which is used to undertake programs until the fund runs out. Imagine that yearly decisions are undertaken; a decision plan is such that it is only undertaken if it is optimal under the situation described below and will be followed through unless the situation changes drastically. Since we allow no uncertainty here, all decisions are final. That is, the optimal course of actions is completely decided for the fund from time zero on; no decision will be revised for the fund in question that is available at time zero.

We can ask at what yearly rate should the eradication program proceed and for what disease. We show that answers to these two questions depend critically on what the burden is at the outset. We take into account that the eradication program requires cumulative effort and that there are stages of development. At any given stage, the society may want to limit its effort because diminishing returns to scale are likely to set in at each period.

Imagine that there is a multiple number of diseases than can be eradicated. The benefit is measured in terms of reduction in burden, and due to the benefit in perpetuity, it is the same for each disease. We develop a simple model of optimal effort level for eradication. Let the total level of successful activity required for the completion of the eradication project be denoted as A. At any given point, $z(t)$ is the accumulated successful activity — eradication production — at time t. Any effort level generates successful activity toward eradication according to $x^{1/2}$; this can be thought of as defining the technology. The society values eradication at B, infinity, and for each year effort enhances production according to

$$z'(t) = x(t)^{1/2}, \tag{6.2}$$

where ' indicates first derivative. Effort level is a cost to the society. Assume that the burden during the period of development is positive in every period or that the total burden during the period rises as the length of research time increases. It is also different for each disease. We simplify by noting that the effect of the total burden prior to eradication is $2T(D)^2$, where T is the duration of the eradication program and D is the burden; and the cost to society is convex.[3] The effect of burden can capture the cost of control program.

With the above scenario, we obtain the following problem:

---

[3] $D(T)$ is the total burden and $D'(T) > 0$ would be consistent with all the results obtained in the section. The formulation here is intended to simplify algebra.

$$\max{}_{x(t)} \; B - 2D^2T - \int_0^T e^{-rt}x(t)dt \qquad \text{subject to}$$

$$z(0) = 0, \; z(T) = A, \tag{7.3}$$

where T denotes the time of completion (to be determined). This problem can be seen as a function of $z(t)$ and the derivative of $z(t)$ with respect to t, $z'(t)$:

$$\max{}_{z'(t)} \; B - 2D^2T - \int_0^T e^{-rt}z(t)^2 dt \qquad \text{subject to}$$

$$z(0) = 0, \; z(T) = A.$$

This solution is formulated as a classical calculus of variations problem. We want to determine the time of completion and, once that has been determined, we can obtain an effort level. It can be shown that this problem yields two roots as a solution for T, only one of which unambiguously yields the result that the optimal time depends negatively on the burden and not at all on B. Further, our intuition is proven correct in that we can claim the relation between T and the burden is unambiguously negative. Once T is determined one can solve for the optimal effort $x(t)$. Hence, the burden during the development period determines the speed at which the vaccine should be developed (see Appendix). The greater the burden, the faster the completion of the eradication program. Hence, we have found a way to prioritize eradication programs.

The society would carry out the exercise above for all eradicable diseases, and then determine the effort level for each of disease. There would be different productivity functions, as well as the cost function. Just in case the technology of eradication is the same for two diseases, we point out that burden and cost of control drive the result. Once T and $x(t)$ are determined, it would undertake these programs until the funds run out; we can easily think of $x(t)$ in terms of monetary cost. Depending on the size of the funds, the administration of many concurrent eradication programs is possible. A point to note is that what was decided at point zero must be followed through in terms of optimal effort each year, no matter that any point in time within the eradication program we may find that the burden from that disease is low.

CONCLUSIONS

As with other proposed health interventions, cost-effectiveness analysis can play an important role in assessing the priority of proposed efforts to eradicate a disease. Eradication efforts, however, present some unique analytical problems related to the near-infinite benefit streams from eradication. The standard solution to this problem in economic appraisal is to discount future health gains at a high rate, typically three percent per year. At such high discount rates, society should only be willing to spend 33 times as much, but no more, to eradicate a disease as compared to curing or preventing it for one year. Arguments in favor of discounting health benefits can and have been widely challenged. If health benefits are not discounted, society should be willing to spend vastly more to eradicate a disease than to manage it for a single year. In fact, following the logic of cost effectiveness, society should be willing to spend nearly all of its health resources on eradication efforts and for similar reasons on health research. In this chapter, we have argued that devoting all current health resources to the improvement of the health of future generations would be to call upon the current generation to make an excessive sacrifice. The only practical solution to the problem of near-infinite benefits is for society to set aside a fraction of health resources that are to be devoted to improving the health of future generations and for the remaining fraction to be spent on the health of the current generation.

How should the funds set aside for improving the health of future generations through eradication and health research be allocated among competing priorities, where many of these competing priorities may have near-infinite benefit streams? Tentatively, we suggest that eradication programs which target diseases with larger causes of burden should be given priority over eradication programs that address smaller causes of burden. Where technology is feasible, the one with the larger burden over a period of time should be given priority.

ACKNOWLEDGMENTS

We would like to thank Kenji Shibuya, Graham Medley, and participants of this workshop for their comments and insights. All remaining errors are ours.

REFERENCES

Acharya, A.K., and C.J.L. Murray. 1997. On discounting benefits on cost-effectiveness analysis. Harvard Center for Population and Development Studies, mimeo.

Arthur, W.B. 1981. The economics of risks to life. *Am. Econ. Rev.* **71**:54–64.

Bloom, D.E., and A.S. Mahal. 1997. Does the AIDS epidemic threaten economic growth? *J. Econometrics* **77**, forthcoming.

Conley, B. 1976. The value of human life in the demand for safety. *Am. Econ. Rev.* **66**:45–55.

Feldstein, M.S. 1964. The social time preference discount and the optimal rate of investment. *Econ. J.* **74**:360–379.

Gold, M.R., J.E. Siegel, L.B. Russell, and M.C. Weinstein. 1996. Cost-effectiveness in Health and Medicine. New York: Oxford Univ. Press.

Jamison, D.T., W.H. Mosley, A.H. Measham, and J.L. Bobadilla. 1993. Disease Control Priorities in Developing Countries. New York: Oxford Univ. Press.

Keeler, E.B., and S. Cretin. 1983. Discounting of life saving and other nonmonetary effects. *Manag. Sci.* **29(3)**:300–306.

Koopmans, T.C. 1965. On the concept of optimal economic growth. In: The Econometric Approach to Development Planning. Amsterdam: North Holland Press.

Lipscomb, J. 1989. Time preference for health in cost-effectiveness analysis. *Med. Care* **27(3)**:S233–S252.

Lipscomb, J., M.C. Weinstein, and G.W. Torrance. 1996. Time preference. In: Cost-effectiveness in Health and Medicine, ed. M.R. Gold, J.E. Siegel, L.B. Russell, and M.C. Weinstein, pp. 214–246. New York: Oxford Univ. Press.

Marglin, S.J. 1963. The opportunity cost of investment. *Qtly. J. Econ.* **77**:95–111.

Mishan, E.J. 1982. Recent contributions to the literature of life valuation: A theoretical approach. *J. Pol. Econ.* **79**:687–705.

Parfit, D. 1984. Reasons and Persons. Oxford: Oxford Univ. Press.

Ramsey, F.P. 1928. A mathematical theory of savings. *Econ. J.* 38:543–559.

Rawls, J. 1971. A Theory of Justice. Cambridge, MA: Harvard Univ. Press.

Redelmeier, D.A., and D.M. Heller. 1993. Time preference in medical decision making and cost effectiveness analysis. *Med. Decision Making* **13**:505–510.

Rice, D.P. 1994. Cost of illness studies: Fact or fiction? *Lancet* **344**:1519–1250.

Sen, A.K. 1961. On optimizing the rate of savings. *Econ. J.* **71**:479–495.

Tengs, T.O., M.A. Adams, J.S. Pliskin, D.S. Safran, and J.E. Siegel. 1994. Five hundred life-saving interventions and their cost-effectiveness. Harvard School of Public Health, Center for Risk Analysis, mimeo.

von Weizsäcker, C.C. 1965. Existence of optimal programs of accumulation for an infinite time horizon. *Rev. Econ. St.* **32**:85–104.

Weinstein, M.C., and W.B. Stason. 1977. Foundation of cost-effectiveness analysis for health and medical practices. *New Engl. J. Med.* **296(31)**:716–721.

World Bank. 1993. World Development Report. New York: Oxford Univ. Press.

Zeckhauser, R. 1975. Procedures for valuing lives. *Public Policy* **23**:419–464.

APPENDIX: THE SPEED OF ERADICATION

The problem described in the section, HOW TO CHOOSE BETWEEN ERADICATION PROGRAMS (see p. 86), can be written as a classical calculus of variations problem, with free end terminal time. In fact, the determination of the terminal time specifies the time of development. Using the notation above the problem is the following:

$$\max_{z'(t)} B - 2D^2T - \int_0^T e^{-rt} z'(t)^2 \, dt \qquad \text{subject to}$$

$$z(0) = 0, \, z(T) = A.$$

The first step consists of obtaining the Euler condition and the transversality condition. The next step is to simply solve for an integral constant and the terminal time using the two derived equations. The Euler condition is the following

$$-2rz'(t)e^{-rt} + z''(t)e^{-rt} = 0, \qquad \text{(A-1)}$$

which entails

$$z'(t) = Ce^{rt}.$$

Integrating this equation and then incorporating the initial condition, we obtain an expression for *z(t)*:

$$z(t) = \frac{Ce^{rt}}{r} - \frac{C}{r}.$$

Note that $z(T) = A$ is the terminal condition; hence, we write $z(t)$ evaluated at T:

$$z(t) = \frac{C(e^{rT} - 1)}{r} = A,$$

which can be solved for C to obtain:

$$C = \frac{Ar}{e^{rT} - 1}. \tag{A-2}$$

The transversality condition is obtained for free terminal horizon:

$$2Ce^{rT} = -2D^2,$$

solving for C, we obtain:

$$C = De^{-\frac{rT}{2}}. \tag{A-3}$$

Using (A-2) and (A-3) and letting $\psi = e^{\frac{rT}{2}}$, we obtain a quadratic equation in ψ, where only the positive root seems sensible. Solving for ψ, we obtain:

$$\psi = \frac{Ar + \sqrt{(Ar)^2 + 4D^2}}{2D}.$$

Substituting for ψ, and then solving for T, we obtain:

$$T = \frac{2}{r} \ln \left[\frac{Ar + \sqrt{(Ar)^2 + 4D^2}}{2D} \right].$$

The relation between T and D is negative as can be seen from taking the first derivative with respect to D. It can be shown that the derivative is unambiguously negative since $4D^2 < (Ar)^2 + 4D^2$. Hence the duration in which the eradication takes place is shortened as the current burden is higher.

8

An Economic Perspective on Programs Proposed for Eradication of Infectious Diseases

M. GYLDMARK[1] and A. ALBAN[2]

[1]Novo Nordisk a/s, Krogshøjvej 31, DK-2880 Bagsvaerd, Denmark
[2]Danish Institute for Health Services Research and Development, Copenhagen, Denmark

ABSTRACT

The purpose of this chapter is to discuss the global and regional economic aspects of programs set up to eradicate infectious diseases. The perspective taken is that scarce health care resources should be employed in the best possible way. Options are examined to determine what the best possible use might be. A starting point is to investigate the relevant policy questions attached to eradication: Is there a suitable technique? What are the costs? What are the benefits? Of particular importance is the opportunity cost of using resources on eradication when other health care problems may require more urgent donation of resources.

This chapter presents a generic model for economic evaluation of eradication programs. As there are many different treatment strategies, each depending on the country or region, such a generic model will need modifications to suit each particular strategy.

This article is contextual and should only be viewed as guidance for those wishing to conduct an economic analysis of eradication programs or to initiate further discussion.

INTRODUCTION

Eradication of infectious diseases (for a definition of eradication, see Fenner et al. and Ottesen et al., this volume) has been the focus of much attention since at least the beginning of this century.

Obviously, eradication of a disease, once achieved, is associated with a tremendous (inestimable) benefit. The absence of a threat to animals' or peoples' health is of enormous value, especially if the disease is widespread and highly infectious.

However, there is also a cost associated with eradication efforts. The costs usually arise immediately while the benefits take time to accrue. There are also alternative uses

---

The Eradication of Infectious Diseases
Edited by W.R. Dowdle and D.R. Hopkins © 1998 John Wiley & Sons Ltd.

of resources, and expenditures directed toward eradication may not always represent the best use of efforts and resources. Other purposes may have more immediate importance. Thus, eradication could be postponed to a later stage, once more pressing problems are dealt with and it achieves higher priority. Put simply, there is a time and place for everything — eradication may not have its time just now.

In this chapter, we discuss the relevant economic aspects of eradication strategies for infectious diseases. We do so by considering what the relevant policy question, with respect to the economic aspects of eradication of infectious diseases, might be. Subsequently, we look at the potential methods for answering these questions and the possibility of obtaining the necessary data. However, we limit the scope here to the aspects of technical and allocative efficiency and ignore aspects of equity. These aspects, however, should not be forgotten.

POLICY QUESTIONS

A number of questions seems relevant to ask in order to explore the economic aspects of eradication programs. We pose some of the questions below but do not attempt to answer all of them in this chapter. Some of the questions must be answered by epidemiologists, medical professionals, or other professionals such as sociologists.

1. What diseases are technically feasible to eradicate?
2. What is an eradication program, i.e., are there alternative strategies for eradicating any specific disease, depending on epidemiology, resources available, organization of health care sector, etc.?
3. Is the choice of eradication strategy contingent on certain aspects, i.e., would the choice of eradication strategy be different for different countries or areas?
4. What are the potential costs of eradication, and who bears the costs?
5. What are the benefits of eradication, and who gains from an eradication program?
6. What is the relation between bearers of cost and gainers of benefits?
7. What information is required to study the costs and benefits?
8. How can this information be obtained, and what is the comprehensiveness and validity of the data?
9. What are the alternatives to eradication, i.e., surveillance and control of present (or a lower) level of infection rates?
10. What is the base line cost today, i.e., what does it cost to maintain and control the present infection rates (by country)?
11. What are the incremental costs and benefits in relation to the alternative strategies, i.e., what is obtained from following an eradication strategy compared to a control or elimination strategy?

All of these questions will be necessary to ask and to answer in order to illuminate fully the economic aspects of eradication programs. The tool to explore the answers to all of these questions in a systematic manner would be to apply one of the economic evaluation techniques.

In the following, we briefly describe the available economic tools.

THE ECONOMIC METHODS

Two very important concepts in economic evaluation are the opportunity cost concept and the concept of marginal costs (and marginal benefits).

The essence of the opportunity cost concept is that since resources are scarce (limited), they have alternative uses. The use of a resource for one purpose will prevent its alternative use for other purposes. The benefit forgone from not employing this resource in its alternative use is the opportunity cost.

Obviously a resource spent on eradication of some disease cannot be spent on other useful purposes. The opportunity cost of eradication programs are potentially very high if alternative uses of scarce resources could yield high(er) (health) benefits.

A note in this respect is that even resources ear-marked for eradication and obtained only for this purpose will have opportunity costs, but these may not be easily detectable.

The marginal cost (or benefit) is an equally important concept. It is the extra cost we have to pay for one extra unit of output. In this context, this would mean the extra resources sacrificed in order to move a step closer to the target. Technically, in this case, we are measuring the incremental costs rather than the marginal costs.

Combining the concept of marginal costs (benefits) with the concept of opportunity costs we get the economic mantra: the opportunity cost at the margin. What do we sacrifice to achieve one more unit of our outcome measure, i.e., what other benefits do we have to sacrifice to achieve one more unit of what we are aiming at achieving in the eradication program?

The possible economic evaluation methods that could be applied to study the above aspects in a systematic way could be the cost-benefit analysis (CBA) or the cost-effectiveness analysis (CEA). A special case of the CEA is the cost-utility analysis (CUA). The advantages of the CUA is that the outcome measure is preference-weighed. An additional advantage is that the measure encompasses both the length and quality of life, and can thus be used to measure the effects of all kinds of health care programs. This is possible because of the common denominator used to compare across interventions and programs. In the context of developing countries, DALYs (disability adjusted life years) are often used as common denominator. The DALY is a measure of effect, but it does not take peoples' perceptions of some health states being less preferred to others into account. In practice, this means that someone (a decision maker or expert group) decides the values attached to the treatment of the different diseases.

The CBA has substantial theoretical underpinning, while there has been some dispute about the theoretical foundation for CEA and CUA (Birch and Gafni 1991; Garber and Phelps 1996). All three types of economic evaluation are, however, widely

| Costs − Avoided Cost = Net Costs | ~ | Benefit = Willingess to Pay |

$$\Rightarrow \quad \frac{\text{Benefit}}{\text{Net Cost}} \geq 1$$

Figure 8.1 The cost-benefit principle.

recognized as pragmatic tools for assessing the economic efficiency aspects of a decision problem (Sugden and Williams 1988).

In relation to economic evaluation, it is important that the choice of evaluation method reflect the questions posed.

If one wishes to know whether "it pays to carry out an eradication program," then the relevant economic evaluation method should be the CBA. In the CBA, every cost and benefit is measured in terms of money (or at least the same unit). According to cost-benefit theory, the net cost of a program should be calculated. The net cost of the program should then be compared to the value attached to the program by the decision makers or target population (i.e., users, non-users, potential users and the nonpotential users). It is then possible to judge whether people find it worthwhile to carry out the program. In some cases, peoples' valuation may be unnecessary as the net cost is negative, i.e., it pays by itself to carry out the program. This principle is illustrated in Figure 8.1.

CEA and CUA are able to answer questions like: which eradication program achieves most of our goal for the resources available, or how do we achieve our goal with a minimum use of resources?

Before we start analyzing, it is therefore essential to pose the right questions and then tailor the economic analysis to the questions we want to address. Another important aspect of economic evaluation is that the perspective for the analysis must be clear.

According to welfare economic theory and the CBA, the appropriate viewpoint (or perspective) for the analysis is the society. However, we have no clear definition of what the society is. Normally, according to textbook welfare economics, the society is confined to the population of a country at a certain time (within a generation) (see e.g., Mishan 1990). If, in this context, the society in mind is the global population for many generations ahead, this would mean a global perspective with an infinite time frame. We would then be moving close to (or perhaps already surpassing) the limits of what economic theory can do.

However, economic evaluations are usually conducted as pragmatic decision-aiding tools, and thus more relevant (for the decision context) perspectives can be adopted.

The relevant perspective for an economic evaluation of an eradication program could therefore be one or more of the following:

- the patient
- the health care sector
- the public sector
- the country

- a region
- the global perspective.

A final aspect of economic evaluation is that these methods are by nature static. They give a snapshot impression of the world as it is now; however, the results may be irrelevant as soon as the underlying assumptions change — and this may happen very quickly.

Having posed these warnings about the abilities of economic evaluation, we proceed to study the underlying assumptions and data for an economic evaluation of eradication programs.

WHICH DISEASES MAY BE ERADICATED?

This question is technical. What techniques are available for eradication of the respective diseases? A proposed list of eradicable and potentially eradicable diseases can, for example, be found in the World Bank Report from 1993 and the International Task Force for Disease Eradication (CDC 1993).

One interesting aspect to note about the eradicable diseases is that the number of people affected is relatively low compared to other infectious diseases; from the number of affected people, the number of deaths are also relatively low compared to other illnesses. This gives an idea about the marginal benefits and the possible opportunity costs. Since the incremental cost by experience increases as harder-to-reach populations are included, opportunity costs may be quite high when resources are devoted to the eradication of a disease. This means that potentially greater benefits could be achieved if the resources were directed to alternative uses.

Before conducting economic evaluations, it is advisable to sift through the list of possible candidates for eradication. This means that economic evaluation is only relevant if the eradication program fulfils a number of preconditions to deem it generally acceptable and feasible. Technical ability is one precondition for eradication. Other preconditions could be:

- The condition should be an important health problem (somehow measured as the disease burden, although this can be problematic).
- There should be an acceptable intervention (e.g., vaccine or other).
- Infrastructure for conducting the intervention should be available (or possible to make available).
- There should be a suitable test or examination for surveillance.
- The test/intervention should be acceptable to the target population.
- The natural history of the disease should be known and understood.
- There should be an policy, acceptable at least on a national level, on how to carry out the intervention.
- The costs of case finding/intervention should be balanced in relation to the possible expenditure on medical care as a whole.

- The health information system should be able to record surveillance data (before and after the intervention).

The above list is a modified version of the European Council recommendations on screening programs (Griffiths and Ruitenberg 1987). Such a list could be further developed for use in selecting eradication programs as candidates for economic evaluation.

Another possibility is to look at the recommendations put forward by Perez Yekutiel (1981). His recommendations are listed in the Appendix. The purpose of the list is to deselect infectious diseases and programs that are not likely to work (achieve the goal) for social, ethical, technical or other reasons.

WHAT IS AN ERADICATION PROGRAM?

Apart from giving a workable definition of eradication (see Fenner et al., and Ottesen et al., both this volume), the question is relevant from the angle: What alternative eradication programs are available, what is the relative cost-effectiveness of these alternative programs, and will the programs vary by country?

Before embarking on an economic evaluation, it is important to identify all possible programs that may lead to the desired goal. To complicate matters, however, possible or viable programs may not be the same for all countries; the relative cost effectiveness may also differ across countries. The preferred strategy may therefore not be the same in Algeria as in Nepal. Assessing global strategies could be a potentially wasteful idea and may also be the reason why the desired goal is not achieved (as the assessed strategy was not viable in some countries).

The choice of an eradication strategy is contingent on a number of issues: epidemiology; the organization, financing and structure of the health care system; accessibility of services; local habits; and/or relative prices.

WHAT IS THE POTENTIAL COST OF AN ERADICATION PROGRAM, AND WHO ARE THE BEARERS OF COSTS?

The resources necessary to carry out an eradication program are obviously many, especially when seen from a global perspective. In addition, resource use depends on the disease, the chosen (alternative) strategies, the countries, their health care systems and practices, and the underlying epidemiology.

Resource use components should be identified and measured in a realistic manner. The following potential costs of an eradication program might be relevant to consider:

1. Direct Costs
   - Overall coordination on a worldwide scale; this means manpower, research, monitoring, evaluation, and information
   - Continuous monitoring of the situation on a global scale

- Country-specific coordination of the routine interventions and any campaigns, "mop-ups," etc.
- Country surveillance for a period after the goal of eradication is achieved, especially if the goal is not achieved in all countries at the same time
- Country-specific information activities
- Production of means for eradication
- Employment of means for eradication, e.g., manpower, equipment, etc.
- Resources spent by the patients or family
- Investment in equipment, buildings, etc.
- Training

2. Indirect Costs
   - Loss of productive time due to the intervention (including travel time)

3. Intangible Costs
   - Any anxiety or stress not measurable as a health outcome, e.g., the thought of intruding in the ecological system.

Each unit of resource used should be affixed a unit price. This unit price should reflect the opportunity cost of that resource. The (free competition) market price is the theoretically correct unit price; however, market prices may not always be obtainable or are often distorted and unreliable.

Finding appropriate prices thus often poses a severe obstacle to producing reliable cost estimates for economic evaluations.

The bearers of costs of eradication programs are multiple and appear at different levels of society. Some of the surveillance costs may be borne by the developed world, but otherwise the costs seem to be borne by the developing countries, where the infectious diseases are most prevalent (again depending on the disease).

The less efficient the health care system is, the more — all other things equal — expensive the eradication program will become; wastage will be higher and compliance lower. To reach the target, marginal costs will have to increase as we move towards eradication.

To identify the bearers of the costs it is necessary to obtain the estimated cost figures for the different components by country or region, adjust these for any differences in time, etc., and calculate the aggregated cost by category. Such categories could be: (1) industrialized countries, (2) middle income countries, and (3) low income countries. The cost pattern by category could then give an idea of the relative bearers of costs. The information is important if related to the distribution of benefits. In case there is a mismatch between the bearers and gainers, there is an argument for a redistribution of resources from the gainers to the losers of eradication.

Without having any figures, it is difficult to say exactly what the relative costs would be and who would bear the costs. It is important, however, that the incremental or marginal costs should serve as the basis for estimation. For developed countries, the marginal cost of adding a new vaccine would be relatively low (the cost of the vaccine itself and some extra time for information and administration), while in a developing country with a poor health care structure, the marginal costs could be relatively high. Cost of mop-ups would also be relatively low in developed countries, but relatively higher in less-developed countries. Delivery might, however, be cheap in a less-developed country and more expensive in the developed world. A number of hypotheses can be proposed with respect to the relative cost burdens, but we need data to verify them.

The calculations presented in the box below help illustrate how the underlying assumptions can influence the relative cost effectiveness of an eradication program.

Cost Effectiveness of Immunization: The Case of Poliomyelitis.

This calculation is based on two model populations: (1) a high mortality population with an assumed life expectancy of 51 years and an infant mortality rate (IMR) of 129/1,000; and (2) a low mortality population with a life expectancy of 64 years and a IMR of 51/1,000.

- The cost of the polio vaccine is considered marginal to other vaccines and is estimated to 3 × US$4 = US$12 per child.
- The number of deaths averted in the high mortality population is set to 170–180 deaths. That is a reduction in IMR by 17–18. In the low mortality population, the corresponding figures are 7 or 8. In addition it is assumed that 50 cases of paralytic polio is averted in each population. This gives a cost per child-death averted of US$670 in high mortality populations and 1,600 in low mortality populations. Including disability cases and assuming a 3% discount rate, the cost per healthy year gained is US$20 and US$42, respectively.
- The numbers are very rough and can only help to illustrate how costs will rise per healthy year gained as the underlying assumptions change and especially how the current situation with respect to risk influence the relative cost-effectiveness of immunization.

Source: Jamison et al. (1993); see also Bart et al. (1996).

WHAT ARE THE BENEFITS OF ERADICATION, AND WHO GAINS FROM AN ERADICATION PROGRAM?

Just as the costs of an eradication program are multiple, so are the benefits. Benefits are also distributed to several gainers, but again the gainers may vary according to which disease we are assessing.

Possible benefits from eradication of an infectious disease include:

1. Direct Benefits
   - Savings in the health care sector due to treatment costs avoided
   - Savings in the health care sector due to prophylactic costs avoided
   - Savings for the patient
   - Savings for the family of patients

- Savings in other sectors of the economy due to reduced morbidity (and mortality)
- Life years gained

2. Indirect Benefits
   - Time benefits (increased productivity/productive time)
3. Intangible Benefits.
   - The absence of a health threat

There are a number of problems in assessing the benefits of eradication programs. First, what forms the basis for comparison? Depending on which alternative treatment scenario is used to compare the eradication program, benefits will achieve different magnitudes. In many cases, the most realistic base for comparison is a control or elimination program. Here, the incremental benefits in switching to an eradication program are mostly in terms of saved prophylactic costs.

In this case, we would not experience a health gain but only a reduced financial "burden" on the health care sector in the future. This financial expense could be appropriately discounted and would reach a finite value that could be compared to the incremental cost of the eradication program.

If the base for comparison is a do-nothing (null) alternative — that may be the likely state of affairs in some countries — then the eradication program will have a most wider spectre of benefits and will include the whole range as written above. In this case, one must consider the issue of discounting health gains (see Acharya and Murray, this volume).

Second, if we want to compare the cost and benefits of an eradication program with the do-nothing alternative, then we need to establish the burden of disease in terms of life years lost due to the disease, as it would be without any interventions. However, as some prophylactic interventions are in place in most countries, it can be hard to assess what the base line would have been.

Third, it has been asserted that the setup and running of eradication programs often have positive external effects in some countries. These external effects include, for instance, the strengthening of the health care sector itself. A strengthened health care sector is better able to take care of other health problems and thus there is a positive spin-off from the eradication program. It is, however, uncertain whether such benefits should be included and, if so, how, since the benefits are not readily measurable.

Given the difficulties in establishing the benefits, it is even harder to say anything about the distribution of benefits until the baseline or relevant alternative is established. It is, however, possible to establish a set of "speculative" hypotheses about the relative value of benefits. For instance, it is possible that the lost savings due to avoided prophylactic measures are relatively high in developed countries, while the gains in terms of life years is large in the less-developed countries. Less-developed countries would probably also have greater savings for the family and for the patients than in the developed countries. Just exactly what the overall balance might be is difficult to say before actual figures are attached to the different components.

In general, however, the primary gainers are probably the patients or the individual, with the community at large as second, and the healthcare sector as the party with least gains (because many are not treated in less-developed countries). This poses a problem in political terms, as decision makers are concerned about budgets and want visible and immediate benefits.

The box below describes the allocation of costs and benefits as tentatively calculated for the successful smallpox eradication program. The calculation shows that the primary gains did not occur in the health sector but rather in other parts of the economy.

Costs and Benefits of Smallpox

The benefits from the eradication of smallpox are considerable. In 1967, 10–15 million people were estimated to be affected by smallpox each year, of which 1.5–2.0 million died. In addition to the saving of lives, eradication has freed up resources for other purposes.

The entire global smallpox eradication program ended up costing about US$300 million over the 13-year period (1967–1979), equivalent to an annual cost of US$23 million. This can be compared to an estimated cost of smallpox in developing countries of more than US$1,070 million. The majority (93%) of this cost was due to loss of production (productivity). The annual cost to industrialized countries was roughly estimated at US$150 million, for U.S.A., and $350 million for all other industrialized countries. In total, the annual cost of smallpox can thus be estimated at more than US$1,350 million for 1967.

Source: Fenner (1988)

INFORMATION AVAILABLE TO CONDUCT AN ECONOMIC EVALUATION OF ERADICATION PROGRAMS

Is it possible to carry out an economic evaluation of eradication programs with the information that is available today? In our experience, health information systems are inadequate in many countries and especially so in the developing countries. The information available about morbidity is thus sparse, or in some cases we will claim so unreliable that it is better not to use it. (An example of this is Nepal, where there is a more than 100% vaccination coverage according to aggregated statistics. The local situation shows quite a different situation, and the actual vaccination coverage is impossible to estimate from the existing records [Onta, unpublished]).

Some of the most crucial pieces of information are simply lacking or of poor quality. It is therefore difficult to judge the opportunity costs of eradication strategies as we do not know what would otherwise have been achieved in terms of reduced mortality and morbidity.

Other information, such as cost of manpower, is also difficult to assess, since the salaries paid in the public sector do not often reflect the opportunity cost of labor.

The cost of the actual means of eradication, the vaccine, or necessary equipment or consumables may have a market price, but this is not even always the case.

Technical Aspects

In addition to identifying costs and benefits, there are a number of technical aspects to take into account when conducting an economic evaluation. We will mention three of these here; for a discussion on the subject of disease modeling, please refer to Medley et al. (this volume).

Time Frame

The first aspect involves chosing a *time frame* for the analysis. This is important as the inclusion of cost components and benefits depend upon the chosen time frame of the analysis. With respect to global disease eradication, the time frame should be fairly long. Even after the last case of the target disease has been detected, it is necessary to continue monitoring to ensure that the disease has really been eradicated. Time frames longer than a generation may therefore be necessary, although the choice will depend on the disease and eradication strategy chosen.

As such, the benefits of global eradication programs can be infinite, as a potential health threat is removed forever. Nonetheless, it is uncertain whether a reduction in overall mortality is actually achieved if we remove one health threat. The result may be that the mortality rate remains constant over the long time frame, and that people die from other diseases instead. This is the problem with partial analysis.

Operating with an infinite time frame does not make sense in practice. From a practical point of view, very long time frames pose political problems as benefits occur in the future while costs are immediate. Politicians have a habit of wanting instant results, and projects with more immediate benefits are generally preferred to projects with longer time spans. In addition, it can be difficult to commit resources for extended periods of time.

If a program fails or stops prematurely, costs have been invested but benefits never reaped. It is therefore natural that decision makers find it hard to agree to very long-term projects.

Discounting

When projects have very long time frames, the issue of *discounting* assumes great importance. Results are generally very sensitive to the choice of discount rates. It will most likely be inappropriate to assume the same discount rate across countries, but using different discount rates will pose a problem to comparability of costs and benefits across countries. The choice of discount rate is thus very important, just as the choice of discounting method is.

It is important that both costs and benefits are discounted. Some studies do not discount health benefits. The theoretical assertion behind this is that the value of health today is the same as value of health tomorrow. Theoretically and technically there are, however, good reasons for discounting health benefits as well (Johannesson 1992). Discounting health benefits has been advocated as good economic practice in all guidelines on economic evaluation (Canada 1994; Australia 1996; Gold et al. 1996). If we can accept to discount health effects, then the problem of infinite benefits is removed since discounting converges the stream of benefits into a finite measure (see Acharya and Murray, this volume).

Since results are so sensitive to the choice of discount rate, we recommend that a sensitivity analysis be carried out for several values of this parameter. In general, sensitivity analysis should be carried out for all parameters where the underlying assumptions are vague, or when the potential impact on the result may be great.

Comparability

Another technical note on the conduct and use of economic evaluations has to do with *comparison of data* and the use of data and evaluation results across countries. The first very basic thing to do when comparing results across countries is to convert costs (and benefits if measured in monetary units) into a common currency and refer them to the same year. However, simple exchange rates do not give a sufficient basis for comparison and purchasing power-adjusted exchange rates (parities), or PPPs, should be used instead. For some countries, health-specific PPPs already exist, but these are flawed and not really appropriate in this context, where a large part of the gains and costs may lie outside the health sector.

Even after adjusting for differences in currency and year of evaluation, there may be tremendous problems in comparing results of economic evaluations across countries. The problems relate to differences in choice of model and differences in relative prices. A program that proves cost effective in one country may not do so in another if the relative prices are significantly different.

CONCLUSION

This chapter expels some of the problems connected with providing evidence in favor or against eradication programs. We propose that economic evaluation of eradication programs be used to study the problem in depth. Through systematic use of economic evaluation, it is possible to uncover the efficiency aspects of eradication programs. This is one step towards better-informed decision making.

Although global eradication of one or more infectious diseases is a covetable goal to achieve, it is associated with sacrifices. These sacrifices may far outweigh the benefits of achieving the goal. A systematic analysis of associated costs and benefits therefore seems advisable before advocating the eradication of infectious diseases. We may win the war, but loose the peace since the sacrifices where too big.

The commitment to eradication programs should be substantial and global as the invested resources otherwise are partly wasted. It is not difficult to imagine the hesitation of decision makers when committing large amounts of resources for long periods of time to a goal that may not be achieved due to unrest or other incidences in other parts of the world.

REFERENCES

Australian Commonwealth. 1992, 1996. Guidelines for the pharmaceutical industry on preparation of submission to the pharmaceutical benefits advisory committee. Canberra: Australian Government Publication.

Bart, K.J., J. Foulds, and P. Patriarca. 1996. Global eradication of poliomyelitis: Benefit cost analysis. *Bull. WHO* 35–45.

Birch, S., and A. Gafni. 1991. Cost-effectiveness/utility analysis: Do current decision rules lead us to where we want to be? Centre for Health Economics and Policy Analysis, McMaster University, Canada.

Canadian Coordinating Office for Health Technology Assessment. 1994. Guidelines for economic evaluation of pharmaceuticals. Canada 1st ed. Ottawa Ont.

CDC (Centers for Disease Control and Prevention). 1993. Recommendations of the International Task Force for Disease Eradication. *Morbid. Mortal. Wkly. Rep.* **42 (RR–16)**:1–38.

Fenner, F., D.A. Henderson, I. Arita, Z. Jezek, and I.D. Ladnyi. 1988. Chapter 31: Lessons and benefits. In: Smallpox and Its Eradication. Geneva: WHO.

Gold, et al. 1996. Cost-effectiveness in Health and Medicine. Washington, D.C.: U.S. Dept. of Health and Human Services.

Jamison, et al. 1993. Disease Control Priorities in Developing Countries (World Bank Book). Oxford Medical Publications.

Griffiths, D.A.T., and E.J. Ruitenberg. 1987. Preventive screening of adults. An evaluation of methods and programs. Maisonneuve, Paris: Council of Europe.

Johannesson, M. 1992. On discounting of gained life years in cost-effectiveness analysis. *Intl. J. Techn. Asses. Health Care* 359–364.

Mishan, E.J. 1988. Cost benefit analysis. London: Unwin Hyman.

Sugden and Williams. 1988. The principles of practical cost benefit analysis. Oxford: Oxford Univ. Press.

Yekutiel, P. 1981. Lessons from the big eradication campaigns. Round table. *World Hlth. For.* **2(4)**:465–490.

APPENDIX: RECOMMENDATIONS FOR UNDERTAKING AN ERADICATION PROGRAM

Precondition 1 There should be a control measure that is completely effective in breaking transmission, simple in application, and relatively inexpensive.

Precondition 2 The disease should have epidemiological features facilitating effective case detection and surveillance in the advanced stages of the eradication program.

Precondition 3 The disease must be of recognized socioeconomic importance, national or international.

Precondition 4 There should be a specific reason for eradication, rather than control, of the disease.

Precondition 5 There should be adequate financial, administrative, manpower and health service resources

Precondition 6 There should be the necessary socioecological conditions.

Source: Yekutiel (1981)

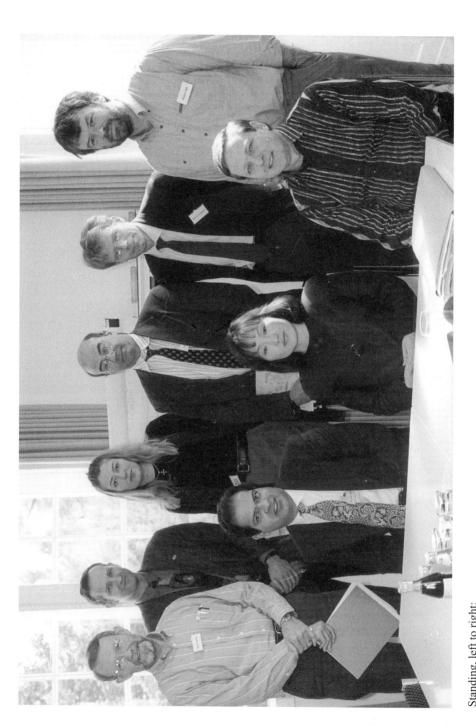

Standing, left to right:
Alan Hinman, Bernhard Schwartländer, Marlene Gyldmark, Ron Waldman, Bruce Aylward, Rob Hall
Seated, left to right:

9

Group Report: What Are the Criteria for Estimating the Costs and Benefits of Disease Eradication?

R.G. HALL, Rapporteur

A.K. ACHARYA, R.B. AYLWARD, M. GYLDMARK,
A.J. HALL, A.R. HINMAN, A. KIM,
B. SCHWARTLÄNDER, R.J. WALDMAN

INTRODUCTION

The decision to eradicate an infectious disease requires judgments on a wide variety of issues. Judgments have to be made on the technical feasibility of eradication, the epidemiology of the condition, the costs and benefits of eradication, and social and political factors. Ethical judgments have to be made on the possible extinction of a species of life and on the impact of eradication and of eradication programs on different societies throughout the world. Moreover, it is unlikely that data of high quality will be available to support rational consideration of all these issues, and further judgments will have to be made regarding the validity and reliability of data, and whether new data will have to be obtained.

Eradication programs consume very considerable resources that could be used for other purposes. An economic analysis allows evaluation of this opportunity cost and is therefore a useful component of decision making.

Economic considerations may help to clarify the following issues:

- Is the use of resources in an eradication program preferable to their use in a nonhealth project?
- Is the use of resources in an eradication program preferable to their use in alternative health interventions?
- Is eradication preferable to continuing control of the condition?

The Eradication of Infectious Diseases
Edited by W.R. Dowdle and D.R. Hopkins © 1998 John Wiley & Sons Ltd.

- Is eradication of this condition preferable to eradication of other eradicable conditions?
- Should eradication of this condition be conducted concurrently with eradication of another condition or should the programs be sequential? If so, should there be an interval between programs?

All these judgments necessitate an evaluation of the costs and benefits of the eradication program(s) and of alternative uses of resources. Many of the costs and benefits of eradication programs have been outlined by Gyldmark and Alban (this volume).

We adopt a definition of eradication that has a global perspective (see Ottesen et al., this volume), and this must clearly also be the view taken in a judgment on whether an eradication program is a "good" use of resources. Despite the global nature of disease eradication, the distribution of costs and benefits will almost certainly vary by region, nation, community, and by group within a community. An analysis of costs and benefits which considers the perspectives of all these entities is both part of a global view and an important element in the political consensus essential to eradication.

Another important perspective relates to time. The target date for eradication of an infectious disease, including certification, will usually be within twenty years of the decision to commence the program, and this effectively determines the time over which costs will be incurred. However, the major attraction of eradication is that benefits then continue to accrue in perpetuity. This presents a particular challenge to traditional economic analysis, as is discussed both by Acharya and Murray (this volume) and below.

We close with some recommendations for how consideration of costs and benefits may assist in the decision-making process and specifically what further research is needed to maximize this usefulness.

ISSUES IN THE ALLOCATION OF RESOURCES

The need for economic analysis of a project, including a proposal to eradicate a disease, relates to two principles:

1. Economic resources (e.g., capital) are scarce.
2. Economic resources may be transferred across sectors.

These principles imply that economic resources should be allocated in a manner which maximizes net benefits to a society or an economy as a whole. In particular, public investment should be justified such that the social value of output due to the investment (e.g., goods and services) exceeds the aggregated value of individual production.[1]

---

[1] This would occur when there is "market failure." In an ideal market; the social value of such goods is the same as the sum of subjective values to individuals.

Public goods and services produce positive externalities. Following this concept, most government investment has been concentrated in sectors such as water supply, transport infrastructure, power, post, education, and health projects.

Outputs produced by these projects can be classified into traded and nontraded goods and services. For projects that produce traded goods and services, economic evaluation can be conducted by comparing costs with benefits in terms of units of constant monetary value (e.g., constant dollars). The value of these traded goods and services is set through the market mechanism of demand and supply. Therefore, selection of the most economically profitable among alternative projects, by using net present value (NPV) and/or economic rate of return (ERR) measures, is relatively straightforward.

On the other hand, a primary output of the health sector is nontraded goods and services, where consumption is equal to production. The standard literature on project evaluation takes nontraded goods and services into account by modifying the prices at which project outputs are valued, with price capturing the net effect or benefit of project output on total market output. However, monetary units may not be the most appropriate way of expressing the value of health benefits, and there is reluctance by many to use prices to value outputs such as lives saved. On the other hand, the valuation of health benefits in monetary terms does allow the comparison of projects in nonhealth and health sectors. Usually, prices are appropriate weights to allow the aggregation of disparate inputs and outputs and thus to derive a single number as a measure of a project's profitability.

In the health sector the improvement of health is the prime objective and measures of health outcomes would be appropriate for evaluation of different health projects. However the use of such measures, DALYs (disability-adjusted life years) or QALYs (quality-adjusted life years) is not without controversy. In addition, the human capital approach, which values improved health outcomes in terms of positive economic benefits, such as enhanced production and/or income-generating capacity, provides another useful way for assessing positive health outcomes.

The human capital approach may be used to delineate a lower bound for an estimate of the cost of the effects of a disease. The true cost of a disease will be greater, since, in addition to the loss of production (the loss of human capital), there is a further loss to society due to the ill health caused by the disease. Society places a value on health in its own right. Despite the exclusion of this loss from consideration, the human capital approach may show a project to be worthwhile. Further, the human capital approach can be useful to show that a health project is as equally profitable as projects in other sectors, given transferability of resources across sectors and the increasing scarcity of public resources.

Any method of valuation of costs and benefits chosen should be considered as somewhat arbitrary, treated tentatively, and examined carefully to ensure that outputs are not sensitive to implicit assumptions.

Eradication of a disease, by definition, demands a global perspective to an economic analysis of the eradication proposal. Theoretically, all countries would receive an infinite stream of benefits from infectious disease eradication, since anyone in any country is at some risk, however small, of the infection over time. The benefit that an eradication program yields, without discounting of future health outcomes, would then be infinite for every country and society.

There will be a differential burden of costs (financially, or in terms of opportunity cost) between countries to complete the components of the eradication program within their borders. An uneven distribution of costs and benefits across countries may result in costs outweighing benefits (for the present generation) of some countries. However, eradication programs yield benefits that can be considered an international public good, and elimination of a disease in every country is eventually required to achieve eradication. One country's elimination task is therefore the business of all other countries. Present generations in the richer countries can afford greater sacrifices in terms of present consumption than can poorer countries. Thus, just as graduated income tax can be imposed on higher income earners to bear a greater cost of parks, national defense, etc., so can richer countries bear a greater proportion of the financial cost of eradication programs. After successful global eradication programs there may be inequities in financial savings, which tend to accrue more to wealthier countries. Wealthier countries bear the bulk of the costs of programs to control the disease and thus most benefit from the ability to cease control efforts. In these countries the risk of disease tends to be assigned a higher social value and consequently elimination is a higher priority. In many developing countries, diseases targeted for global eradication are not considered to be particularly important, especially when considered alongside other health problems which are responsible for much greater levels of incapacitation and death.

Furthermore, since an infectious disease eradication program is usually undertaken within a generation, the costs will burden the present generation more than future generations. The eradication program may put a very large cost burden on the present generation, if the disease has a low burden of illness and/or the cost of the program is high. Implementation of an eradication program may divert resources away from other health interventions or even from economic growth. In this case the present generation may not wish to undertake the program.

TYPES OF ECONOMIC ANALYSIS

Implicit in the decision to attempt to eradicate a disease is the idea that the benefits exceed the costs. There are issues of the most appropriate type of economic analysis required to assess the merits (in terms of costs and benefits) of a disease eradication program. The nature of the analysis undertaken should be dependent on the questions needing answers. Current formal economic analytical techniques are not ideally suited to eradication programs. There is, for example, lack of agreement on how to handle future benefits and costs, particularly long-term effects ("effects in perpetuity"), and there is disagreement as to whether and how to discount future effects. Economic analyses should be performed and published showing future effects both discounted and not discounted.

Cost-benefit and cost-effectiveness (including cost-utility) analyses may both contribute to a decision on launching a disease eradication initiative. Of these techniques cost-effectiveness analysis appears to be the most useful, in that the outcome is expressed in health terms and thus it allows evaluation of disease eradication when compared with other projects in the health sector. It follows that, using this technique, a comparison of health and nonhealth projects, and therefore rational decisions on allocation of resources between sectors, cannot be made.

Past experience has shown that the decision to embark on an eradication program has not been made with regard to competition for resources across sectors. A cost-effectiveness analysis comparing the option of disease control (to a specified level) with the option of disease eradication, and an analysis of the marginal costs and benefits of proceeding from a specified level of control to eradication, would provide decision makers with a useful assessment of the economic worth of a disease eradication initiative.

Economic analyses should clearly state their objectives, the assumptions used, the time horizon, estimates of confidence in the results, and the perspectives taken, with the aim of transparency for the reader. Any formal economic analyses undertaken should take a global perspective but should be based on national and regional-level analyses. The time frame to consider is problematic but should include, at least, the period of the eradication activity and the 10–30 years ("one generation") after eradication has been achieved and intervention to control the disease has been ceased.

One alternative methodology intended to overcome some of the difficulties in the choice of which agent to eradicate is the use of burden of disease (see Acharya and Murray, this volume).

COSTS AND BENEFITS OF GLOBAL ERADICATION PROGRAMS

The costs and benefits from global eradication programs can be grouped into two categories:

- Direct effects, since after eradication of a condition no disease-specific morbidity or mortality due to the eradicated disease will ever occur, and control programs can be ceased; and
- Consequent effects on the health care system, which would traditionally be classified as an externality in economic analysis.

For polio eradication, for example, this means that there will be no deaths from polio, and no need for treatment and rehabilitation services. The global financial savings on vaccine costs alone are estimated to be on the order of US$ 1.5 billion per year. There are also intangible benefits, including increased personal and family security due to the removal of the threat of infection from polio, and an improved image and morale of public health programs and personnel.

Although the costs saved due to eradication of infectious diseases can seem very large in absolute terms, they represent only a small proportion of the overall health budget and even a small proportion of the costs of related programs which will have to continue. For example, immunization against other vaccine-preventable diseases continues after the eradication of smallpox.

Eradication of a particular disease may greatly benefit those who are at greatest risk, but may have limited impact on the global burden of disease and ill-health. Neither smallpox nor poliomyelitis eradication, for example, contributes (or will contribute) substantially to a reduction in the global burden of illness — both incidence and disease-specific mortality and disability rates are relatively low. Crude and age-specific mortality rates are only minimally affected by their eradication, if at all. However, eradication programs can contribute to the attainment not only of benefits directly due to the eradication of the target infection, but also of an extended "package" of benefits which, if realized, could have an important impact on health outcomes in developing countries. This other category of benefits may be conceptualized as "improvements to the effectiveness of health care." The production of these benefits, in economic terms, "positive externalities," was a principal objective of the polio elimination program in the Americas. Conversely, in many situations, especially in countries with relatively weak health infrastructures, eradication programs can come into competition with the development of other health care programs. Although it would not be fair to require that eradication programs bear the entire burden of health system development, they do represent an important opportunity to make a substantial contribution to the strengthening of health systems, as has been amply documented in the Americas by the polio elimination efforts.

Eradication programs must operate within a relatively short time frame to generate and maintain the interest and to secure the resources which allow them to be completed. The attainment of eradication will invariably come before health infrastructure development can be completed. But in the rush to reach zero incidence, attention should continue to be focused on attainment of the entire benefits package.

Eradication of a disease leads to a health improvement which persists forever, and the importance of this persistence should not be understated. However, eradication does not occur in a vacuum and such programs should contribute to the realization of an entire package of benefits (see discussion by Foege, this volume).

INTANGIBLE COSTS AND BENEFITS

Although relatively objective criteria exist for the valuation in quantitative terms of many aspects of eradication initiatives, the measurement of some costs and benefits is complicated by their subjective nature. While intangible costs and benefits are not unique to eradication initiatives, they may constitute a substantial aspect of the overall impact of the program. An attempt should therefore be made to at least identify these intangibles and assess their magnitude.

Examples of the intangible effects of eradication initiatives include their impact on the improved motivation, morale, and self-esteem of health workers. Conversely, the sense of urgency which accompanies an eradication initiative may inadvertently result in very large demands on an overworked health worker, resulting in a loss of motivation. Such intangible effects are not limited to individuals, and may apply, positively or negatively, to large parts of the health care system.

While it may be possible to identify many of the intangible effects of an eradication program before implementation, the impact of some effects may be very difficult to predict. There may be, for example, an impact of an eradication program on human rights. The inappropriate enforcement of eradication strategies could contravene the rights of individuals or societies. There may be value conflicts with deeply held religious or other beliefs.

Some of the impacts of health interventions which may be measurable in a national setting may pose particular problems in a global eradication initiative, due to wide variations in the valuation of such costs and benefits in different cultures, or the absence of any data on their value. The pain and suffering due to a disease, or the stigmatization associated with that disease, may be regarded very differently between, and even within, cultures and countries. A similar consideration may be needed for costs incurred in the course of implementing an eradication initiative's strategies.

OTHER DETERMINANTS IN THE DECISION TO EMBARK ON ERADICATION OF A DISEASE

All decisions to eradicate infectious disease involve economic considerations. Typically these reflect issues of the financial costs of eradication programs and future costs to be avoided through eradication. However, economic analyses are only one of the tools employed in the decision to embark on an eradication program. It is important to consider the context within which such decisions are made and the role of economic analysis *vis a vis* other considerations. Economic analyses support, rather than determine, decisions on whether or not to undertake the eradication of an infectious disease.

Economic analysis is dependent on a knowledge of some of the issues listed below, and several will need to be assessed even if no economic analysis is performed. Factors which may be likely to play a decisive role include:

- Technical factors regarding the intervention, such as its efficacy and effectiveness, ease of use, duration of effect, and durability of any effect;
- Operational factors, for example, logistical considerations in implementing the intervention;
- Factors relating to the epidemiological burden of disease, including morbidity and mortality;

- Epidemiological factors, including the cyclicity of the condition (and the possibility of magnified effect if the intervention is carried out during a period of low transmission), the populations most affected, the age at which the condition occurs and the age at which the intervention is effective;
- Financial factors, including the overall direct costs of the program, the availability of resources, and the possibility of attracting "new" resources which were not originally destined for this purpose and would otherwise have been used for other, possibly nonhealth, purposes;
- Social factors, including the awareness and interest of the public at large, the acceptability to the public of the intervention, the possibility of social mobilization, and the degree of community involvement;
- Political factors, since high-level political commitment is essential for eradication programs; and
- Timing, both with respect to the vulnerability of the condition (for example, a disease already under a substantial degree of control or at a low point in its natural cycle) and with respect to the possibility of being able to combine efforts (for example the addition of rubella eradication to a measles eradication effort).

Experience to date suggests that avoidance of future costs of control programs and political support have been among the most important deciding factors in the decision to launch disease eradication programs. The concept of the time to the "break-even point" (that is the point at which savings due to eradication equal expenditure on the eradication program) has proved to be particularly useful as an intuitive way of presenting the future financial savings due to an eradication initiative.

It has been stated that eradication programs represent the ultimate in equity since they provide equal protection to all persons against the disease in question. However, under some circumstances it is possible that eradication programs could increase health inequities in an area if, for example, they draw resources away from other programs which could have had an even greater impact on health. Eradication efforts confer both benefits and costs on other health programs. Many of these effects have been described, but documentation and quantification are inadequate and relevant data should be collected and analyzed.

Because of the close interrelationships between eradication programs and other health programs, eradication goals and activities should be expressed in the context of overall health services and explicit efforts should be taken to maximize the effectiveness of both the eradication and comprehensive health programs (see Foege, this volume).

CONCLUSIONS AND RECOMMENDATIONS

Disease eradication initiatives are unique in public health in that, if successful, they result in a health gain which persists forever. This feature is fundamental, and is a major reason for undertaking such activities. Economic analysis is only one element in reaching decisions on eradication programs, and supports, rather than determines the decision. There are theoretical problems in economic analysis which are specific to eradication, and in particular the future benefits require resolution. Economic analyses of eradication should take a global perspective but analyses at regional and national level form important components of this overall global analysis.

Because of the close interrelationship between eradication programs and other health programs economic analyses should incorporate the costs and benefits resulting from the effects of the eradication program on other health programs.

Presentation of economic analysis should enable the reader to determine the costs, benefits and externalities, direct and indirect. The results of economic analyses should be presented with both discounted and undiscounted health gains.

Research is required:

- On economic methods to deal with the special features of eradication programs which include the infinite time horizon for benefits, the potentially high costs of failure to eradicate the target disease, and the global nature of the program.
- On the costs and benefits of current eradication programs, in particular those related to effects on the health programs in all regions of the world. These include both epidemiological and economic data.
- On the utility of new methods (from Pt. 1 above) and new data (from Pt. 2 above) in the evaluation of current eradication programs.
- To produce good economic analyses of successful and unsuccessful programs already undertaken or underway (malaria, smallpox, poliomyelitis and Guinea worm disease [dracunculiasis]). Such studies would help illustrate the issues involved and clarify methodological problems.

10

Roles for Public and Private Sectors in Eradication Programs

C.A. DE QUADROS[1], A.C. NOGUEIRA[1], and J.-M. OLIVÉ[2]

[1] Special Program for Vaccines and Immunization, Pan American Health Organization, 525 23rd Street NW, Washington, D.C. 20037, U.S.A.
[2] Global Program for Vaccines and Immunization, World Health Organization, 1211 Geneva 27, Switzerland

ABSTRACT

Over the last few years, health systems throughout the world have entered a process of reform that include a high degree of decentralization and downsizing of the public health sector. These processes have brought as a consequence an increased role for private sector institutions involved in providing health care and more participation from local organizations and communities. These trends indicate that the public health sector alone cannot achieve health objectives if there is not a full participation of all sectors of society, including the communities themselves.

This chapter presents the experiences of partnership between the public and private sectors during the initiative that culminated with the eradication of indigenous transmission of wild poliovirus from the Western Hemisphere and the present efforts to eradicate measles from the same region by the year 2000. Inter-agency coordination, under the leadership of the Ministry of Health, was the key for the achievement of a harmonious relationship among several public and private sector organizations that ultimately facilitated the elimination of poliomyelitis and is now advancing the elimination of measles.

The partnerships were important not only for the detailed planning of activities that need to be implemented at the national and local levels, but also for generating political and social will. Through innovative ways, they have increased the ownership of the initiatives and the availability of resources that otherwise were untapped at the national level.

The experiences in the Americas demonstrated that with a high level of political commitment, the public sector can participate in a partnership with private sector organizations to achieve important results that improve the health of the populations. These experiences may be useful for future initiatives for the eradication of infectious diseases.

INTRODUCTION

After inoculating James Phipps with the first smallpox vaccination in 1796, Edward Jenner declared that "this practice will wipe out this scourge from the face of the earth."

The Eradication of Infectious Diseases
Edited by W.R. Dowdle and D.R. Hopkins © 1998 John Wiley & Sons Ltd.

It took almost 200 years for his prediction to became a reality when, in 1977, Ali Maow Maalin was detected with smallpox in Somalia as the last case of naturally occurring infection with the smallpox virus (Fenner et al. 1988).

Poliovirus vaccines were developed in the 1950s, and it took almost 40 years for the certification that poliomyelitis transmission was interrupted in the Western Hemisphere, after the two-year-old Luis Fermin of Peru was diagnosed as the last case of paralytic poliomyelitis due to the wild poliovirus in August, 1991 (Robbins and de Quadros 1997). This disease will also be consigned to history early in the 21st century (Hull et al. 1994).

It remains to be seen how long it will take until the last case of measles is detected somewhere in the world and this major childhood killer is declared eradicated (de Quadros et al. 1996). A vaccine against this disease was introduced in the early 1960s.

These few examples illustrate the gap that exists between the availability of technologies and their full application to the benefit of all humankind. They emphasize the critical role played by the political and social will that needs to be present if the entire population of the planet is to improve its health and welfare through the full utilization of modern technologies and equitable access to basic health services.

Over the last few decades, the public sector[1] has evolved from a very centralized system to a decentralized one, in which local governments are assuming an ever-increasing role. This power sharing between central and local governments has led to joint decisions on funding and implementation of health programs, as well as increased responsibility of local entities in these processes. Central governments still maintain a prominent role in setting national norms and in issues related to regulation and quality control.

As the process of decentralization occurs, there is a downsizing of the public sector and, as a result, an increasing number of organizations, institutions, and individuals from the private sector[2] start playing an important role in policy setting and actual provision of health services. These institutions are mainly represented by nongovernmental organizations both of national and international origin, but also including national and multinational industrial enterprises.

During the years of the global smallpox eradication program, health systems and services in the majority of countries were extremely centralized, and activities were

---

1 Public Sector: all entities that are financed and managed by national, regional, or local governments. This chapter addresses primarily those entities involved with the public health sector. Included in this category are multilateral and bilateral developmental organizations that are financed by governments.

2 Private Sector: all entities that are organized, financed, and managed outside of government responsibility. Included in this category are national and international entities such as private enterprises (e.g., vaccine and drug manufacturers), not for profit and for profit nongovernmental organizations (NGOs) as well as private voluntary organizations (PVOs), religious groups, labor organizations, and local community organizations (e.g., mothers' clubs and volunteers).

implemented almost entirely by the public sector institutions, with limited support from the private sector and international organizations besides the World Health Organization. However, despite this limited participation of the private sector, there were some critical contributions, such as the release of the patent rights for both the bifurcated needle, by Wyeth Laboratories, and for the freeze drying technology rights for the smallpox vaccine, by the Lister Institute. At the field level, local organizations also participated in helping organize communities for ʹvaccination campaigns and surveillance (D.A. Henderson, pers. comm.)

With this background, governments have begun to recognize that they cannot fully meet all health needs of their people by relying solely on public health providers and resources; it is practically impossible to achieve success in disease eradication without a more extensive and full partnership between the public and private sectors as well as with all developmental organizations that collaborate with any given government. Alliances need to be formed between the public health sector, social security systems, and private sector enterprises to achieve national public health objectives. These partnerships are appearing in all countries with varied degree of intensity.

This chapter discusses the critical roles of the public and private sectors in bringing available disease prevention technologies to their full potential by describing the close collaboration between all sectors of society during the successful campaign that eliminated poliomyelitis from the Western Hemisphere, as well as during the recent efforts to eliminate measles from the Americas by the year 2000.

POLIO AND MEASLES ERADICATION INITIATIVES: EXPERIENCES IN THE AMERICAS

In 1985, the Pan American Health Organization (PAHO) launched an initiative to eliminate poliomyelitis from the Western Hemisphere (de Quadros et al. 1992). For this initiative to be successful, it was necessary that (a) all governments be committed to the goal and assign the necessary resources to ensure its success, (b) that all sectors of society become involved, and (c) all international, bilateral, multilateral, and NGOs participate in the process of collaboration with national governments in a coordinated fashion.

Political commitment was achieved through a resolution of the Directing Council of PAHO and on-going discussions between PAHO officials and authorities of the countries involved.

To address the issues related to the relationship between the public and private sector and inter-agency coordination necessary to achieve proper relationship amongst all partners PAHO, the Inter-American Development Bank (IDB), Rotary International, the United Nation's Children's Fund (UNICEF), and the United States Agency for International Development (USAID) joined forces in 1985, to form an Interagency Coordinating Committee (ICC) that, through a memorandum of understanding, pledged to coordinate activities in support of governments, avoiding duplication and competition to maximize their resources. However, this collaboration could only be possible if based on a Regional Plan of Action, which in turn would be reflected in the planning processes of the governments involved. The Regional Plan of Action, prepared by PAHO in consultation with the other partners, called for the creation of an ICC in each country, which would in turn support the national five-year plans of action that outlined the activities to be carried out with identification of the resource requirements for implementation.

The responsibility of the Ministries of Health was to prepare the National Plans of Action (NPA) for the 1987–1992 five-year period to serve as the basic instrument through which the host government, the ICC, and other organizations, including NGOs could participate in a coordinated fashion. They simultaneously permitted national health managers to plan and budget their use of resources in detail, including cost analyses of activities by type (capital/recurrent) and source (national/external).

At the national level and under the coordination of a high-level representative of the Ministry of Health (in many countries the Minister himself/herself), ICCs met regularly to follow up the implementation of planned activities, identify obstacles and revise it accordingly, and prepare the NPA for the next calendar year.

Furthermore, the NPA made it possible to assess the sustainability of national immunization programs within the larger health service infrastructures. The likelihood of financial sustainability, to ensure that adequate personnel and supplies would be available over time, can be measured by the analysis of the NPAs data. For example, in the first five-year plan (1987–1991), 80% of the total cost of US$ 544.8 million invested in 17 countries was covered by national sources and 20% (US$ 113.8) by external sources. During this phase, national resources represented primarily opportunity costs including salaries, facility maintenance, and transportation. The second five-year plan from these countries, 1992–1996, indicates that a total of US$ 774.9 million had been projected, of which nearly 92% was to be provided by national sources and 10% (US$ 61 million) was being sought from external sources. The data shown in Figure 10.1, including the projections for a third five-year period (1997–2001), show the tendency of these expenditures, demonstrating a continued increase in national investments as a result of political commitment that assign high priority to highly cost-effective programs.

From the inception of the polio eradication initiative, particularly after it was realized that the second five -year regional plan would receive a smaller grant from the major grantor to the program (USAID), efforts were made at regional and country levels to increase the partnership with several other organizations, especially national and international private voluntary organizations (PVOs).

Considerable time of international PAHO consultants was dedicated specifically to contact and inform the potential partners of the opportunities for collaboration, to prepare special projects to address this collaboration, and to ensure that ICCs would incorporate these new organizations. As a result of these efforts, an estimated US$3.6 million was added locally during 1992; the first year, the partnership started to expand, and from then on, the participation of NGOs and PVOs has been regularly monitored at national level.

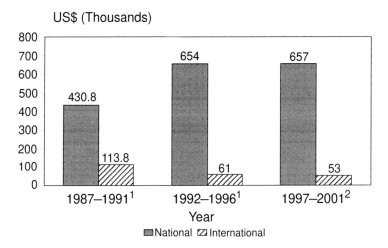

1 Includes polio eradication
2 Includes measles elimination (estimated)

Figure 10.1 National and international expenditures on immunization programs in the Americas, 1987–2001. Source: EPI/PAHO and National Plans of Action.

The continued involvement of high-level public and private sector officials has stimulated the sustained participation of these organizations and other voluntary groups. If properly nurtured, this trend is likely to continue. For example, reports of the 1994 and 1995 ICC meetings held in the various countries of the region show a marked increase in the participation of PVOs in support of immunization programs, that at this stage include the goal of measles eradication (Table 10.1).

An excellent example of public sector commitment is the recent establishment of a budget line for the national immunization activities enacted in the national budget of Guatemala. Similar laws should be enacted in all countries to ensure the permanence of these programs, and PAHO is actively collaborating with legislators in various countries to facilitate this process.

The involvement of nontraditional partners in immunization programs has been extensive and varied. Partners, from PVOs, commercial manufacturers, parliaments and religious groups, baby food manufacturers, soft drink companies, and travel agents, to local organizations and community groups, provided all sorts of collaboration, such as transportation, meals, volunteer staff for vaccination clinics, as well as promotional equipment and media support. They have also participated in training programs, procurement of vaccines, and identification and mobilization of hard-to-reach groups such as indigenous populations. This collaboration was always managed through the ICCs, and their involvement was particularly critical for the implementation of the key strategies for polio eradication, such as organization of national immunization days (NIDs) and mop-up operations, as well as surveillance for acute flaccid paralysis (AFP).

Table 10.1   Number of PVO's collaborating with immunization programs in selected countries, 1994–1995.

COUNTRY	1994	1995
Bolivia	12	53
Dominican Republic	4	8
Ecuador	—	5
El Salvador	42	66
Guatemala	12	7
Honduras	5	20
Nicaragua	4	20
Peru	8	10

Source: EPI/PAHO, and reports of national ICC meetings

One of the major elements for a successful NID is to ensure that proper logistics will secure vaccine availability to all groups of populations and that social communication strategies will convey the appropriate messages to be clearly understood by those supposed to participate in the event, such as the parents of the children that need to be vaccinated and by those who have to report the presence of cases of AFP immediately. The extension of AFP surveillance to the most remote communities was only possible with the involvement of PVOs and NGOs, which often cover remote communities not served by the public health sector. Additionally, in the last stages of polio elimination, when a reward of US$ 100.00 was offered by PAHO to anyone reporting a case of AFP that eventually was confirmed as due to wild poliovirus, a private sector organization in some countries raised this reward to US$ 1,000.00, increasing the attractiveness of AFP reporting. An innovative way of stimulating PVO participation was the use of seed money provided by the mother organization, which in turn generated local fund raising and participation in program activities. In Peru (R. Cardoso, pers. comm.), for example, local Rotary clubs generated funding in excess of 20 times the amount of seed money provided by the centralized Rotary International PolioPlus Program, without counting the in-kind contributions.

Coordination with vaccine manufacturers was also important in terms of ensuring the prompt availability of good quality vaccine at accessible prices. This was achieved by a permanent dialogue with manufacturers and the purchase of the vaccines through a revolving fund that allowed countries to utilize local currencies to purchase their vaccine needs. This revolving fund, administered by PAHO, provided vaccine manufacturers with good estimates of vaccine needs, allowing for the smooth programming of production and capital investments for expansion of production capabilities.

Feedback from the public sector was also fundamental for the adjustment of vaccine composition as was the case with the oral poliomyelitis vaccine. When a polio type 3 outbreak was detected in northeast Brazil in late 1980s, the epidemiological analysis demonstrated that the cause was a low concentration of the poliovirus type 3 in the trivalent oral poliomyelitis vaccine (Patriarca et al. 1988). When this information was passed to the manufacturers there was an almost immediate reformulation of the concentration of this virus type, and the program did not suffer a break in continuity. This was a good model of collaboration and of the prompt response from the private sector in support of the eradication program.

Following the positive experiences with the polio elimination effort, the Plan of Action for Measles elimination also called for international collaboration in support of the program (de Quadros et al. 1992, 1996). Up to this moment there is financial support from multilateral and bilateral agencies, such as USAID, UNICEF, IDB, the Spanish Agency for International Cooperation (AECI), the Swedish International Development Agency (SIDA), the Canadian International Development Agency (CIDA), the Office of International Cooperation of the Netherlands, the French International Health Cooperation, the Japan International Cooperation Agency (JICA), and several NGOs or PVOs. While the collaboration of the external agencies is critical for program success, the bulk of resources is provided by the countries themselves (Figure 10.1).

CONCLUSIONS

The regional initiatives to eliminate poliomyelitis and now to eliminate measles and the ongoing efforts to maintain high immunization coverage levels and control other communicable diseases attests to the impact of well-coordinated approaches. Such approaches can only be implemented once there is national commitment and allocation of the necessary resources to carry on the activities at regional and country level. This continued national and international commitment will be critical for the success of other disease eradication initiatives eventually launched in the future.

From these experiences in the Americas, it is clear that private sector involvement was successful because it was conceived as a partnership that started in a time-limited approach but which eventually became ongoing. The success was in great part due to the very clear and achievable goal of disease eradication, in which the public sector assumed the major responsibility for funding and the leadership in the coordination process as *primus-inter-paris*. On the other hand, the participation of the private sector, particularly the NGOs and PVOs, did not replace the major responsibilities of the public sector, in these cases the Ministry of Public Health, illustrating some of the synergism that builds up with partnerships for disease eradication. While the public sector is critical to generate the political will and harness the needed resources allocated by national budgets, it is necessary that other sectors participate actively in generating the social will which in the final instance will ensure the success of these initiatives.

Another role of the public sector is in the realm of organization of national plans and definition of strategies that need to be implemented uniformly throughout a nation. Even in this respect, the private sector, including the organized groups of society and communities, should participate as early in the process as possible so that there is ownership of the strategies and plans to be implemented. The private sector plays a key role in terms of advocacy and in the maintenance of the political and social will by having easy access to decision makers and community leaders.

Difficulties encountered in the Americas included the initial difficulties of Ministries of Health in accepting the full participation of the private sector, particularly nongovernmental organizations in the process of national planning of activities and in the need for a high degree of recognition of their collaboration. Learning to work together was not always an easy process but it was a constructive one leading to a spirit of achievement and a renewed positive image of both the public health sector, represented by the Ministry of Health and the private sector, represented by the various national and international organizations referred to in this paper. As programs evolved and more experience was gained with joint implementation of such programs, the initial difficulties were overcome and a high degree of efficiency was achieved by these partnerships.

The lessons from the Americas show that commitment to a national goal, with preparation of medium-term plans of action and leadership within participatory ICCs, increases the confidence of the private sector to participate in national and local initiatives that can have substantial impact in the health of the populations. These lessons may be of interest for future disease eradication initiatives.

Questions still remain to be answered about the role of decentralization on the importance and influence of the public health sector, including social security systems, private health care providers, and health insurance groups in the delivery of health care and disease prevention services, including future eradication programs. Analysis of the experiences emanating from countries and regions where decentralization and privatization are more advanced will be critical in helping to define the potential roles and partnerships between the public and private sectors in the coming years.

REFERENCES

de Quadros, C.A., J.K. Andrus, J.M. Olivé, C.G. de Macedo, and D.A. Henderson. 1992. Polio eradication from the Western Hemisphere. *Ann. Rev. Pub. Hlth.* **13**:239–252.

de Quadros, C.A., J.M. Olivé, B.S.Hersh, M. Strassburg, D.A. Henderson, D.B. Bennet, and G.A.O. Alleyne. 1996. Measles elimination in the Americas: Evolving strategies. *JAMA* **275(3)**:224–229.

Fenner, F., D.A. Henderson, I. Arita, Z. Jezek, and I.D. Ladnyi. 1988. Smallpox and Its Eradication. Geneva: WHO.

Hull, H.F., N.A. Ward, B.P. Hull, J.B. Milstein, and C.A. de Quadros. 1994. Paralytic poliomyelitis: Seasoned strategies, disappearing disease. *Lancet* **343**:1331–1337.

Patriarca, P., F. Laender., G. Palmeira, M.G.C. Oliveira, J.L. Filho, M.C. de Souza Dantas, M.T. Cordeiro, and J.B. Risi. 1988. Randomized trial of alternative formulations of oral poliovaccine in Brazil. *Lancet* **1**:429–433.

Robbins, F.C., and C.A. de Quadros. 1997. Certification of eradication of indigenous transmission of wild poliovirus in the Americas. *J. Infec. Dis.* **175 (Suppl. 1)**:S281–S285.

11

Overcoming Political and Cultural Barriers to Disease Eradication

S.O. FOSTER

Visiting Professor, Dept. of International Health, Rollins School of Public Health, Emory University, 1518 Clifton Road, Atlanta, GA 30322, U.S.A.

ABSTRACT

This chapter addresses the political and cultural barriers constraining the effective implementation of eradication strategies assessed as meeting three criteria: (1) address a major cause of morbidity, disability, or mortality; (2) utilize a technical strategy that has the potential to stop transmission and achieve eradication; and (3) have the potential economic benefits that justify the costs of eradication versus the opportunity costs of using those same funds for other development and health priorities.

Utilizing a model portraying elements involved in implementing eradication programs, this article identifies barriers to eradication and strategies useful or potentially useful in overcoming them. Barriers identified through a search of the literature and key informant interviews are categorized into five groups: barriers in vision, barriers in context, barriers in content, barriers in process, and barriers in operations. Eradication program experiences in overcoming these barriers are shared.

INTRODUCTION

Disease eradication strategies have the potential to contribute to long-term improvements in global health and development in a cost-effective manner. Since most diseases targeted for eradication disproportionately affect the rural impoverished poor, eradication initiatives also preferentially address the most needy. Only a few diseases, however, meet the criteria identified by the International Task Force for Disease Eradication (CDC 1993).

The title of this chapter was changed from the proposed "Cultural and Political Factors Determining the Prospects of Eradication" to "Overcoming Political and Cultural Barriers to Disease Eradication." This reformulation evolved from my experience with three of the "eradicable" diseases: smallpox, polio, and measles. The

The Eradication of Infectious Diseases
Edited by W.R. Dowdle and D.R. Hopkins © 1998 John Wiley & Sons Ltd.

smallpox years involved field assignments in Nigeria, Bangladesh, and Somalia (1966–1977). The polio experience focused on epidemiology, the Expanded Program on Immunization (EPI), and child survival in 12 African countries and led to the understanding that polio was a controllable but not an eradicable disease. Results in the Americas (de Quadros et al. 1997) and the progress of poliomyelitis eradication in Asia have altered that perspective. Despite the better than expected progress in the Americas toward measles elimination, I have continuing concerns about the technical feasibility, not the desirability, of global measles eradication (de Quadros et al. 1996; Foster et al. 1993).

METHODS

Four sources were utilized in the preparation of this chapter:

- a review of the literature on disease eradication,
- phone interviews with colleagues[1] involved in past and current eradication programs (malaria, smallpox, dracunculiasis, and measles),
- reflections on the day-to-day experience in implementation of disease prevention, control, and eradication programs in developing countries,
- comments received from participants at the Dahlem Workshop.

ERADICATION FRAMEWORK

Success in eradication requires not only science and technology, but also the disciplines of anthropology, communications, economics, management, politics, and public policy. This complexity is captured, in part, by Walt in her article on policy analysis: "health policy wrongly focuses attention on the content of reform and neglects the actors involved in policy reform (at the international, national, and sub-national levels), the processes involved on developing and implementing change, and the context within which policy is developed" (Walt and Gilson 1994, p. 354). Her schematic representation of these interactions has been adapted to provide the framework for this chapter (see Figure 11.1). The three angles of the triangle reflect the three arenas in which decision makers (Walt uses the term "actors") interact in the formulation of policy. The left side of the triangle conveys the incremental nature of eradication as it expands from local, to regional, to national, to global. It also identifies three key support strategies essential to this expansion: the preparation and distribution of technical guidelines, international assistance of personnel and resources, and regular

---

1 Peter Carrasco, D.A. Henderson, Don Hopkins, Pat Mcconnon, Randy Packard, Ted Trainer, Craig Withers

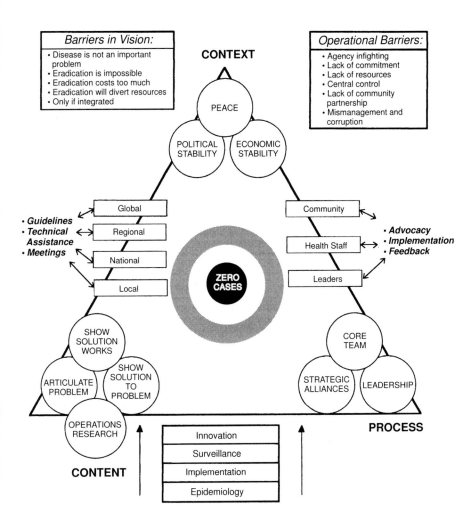

Figure 11.1   Overcoming political and cultural barriers to disease eradication.

meetings to share commitment, experience, and issues. The right side of the triangle portrays the challenge of building the eradication team and co-opting political and health leaders, health staff, and most importantly the community to that team. The bottom of the triangle is made up of four foundation stones essential to all eradication programs: epidemiology, implementation, surveillance, and innovation. The two outside boxes summarize the barriers identified by colleagues queried by telephone. The bulls-eye in the center emphasizes the raison d'etre of eradication: zero cases and the bottom line by which all actions are judged.

BARRIERS IN VISION

Initiating a disease eradication strategy involves not only providing a feasible, logical, affordable operational plan, but also addressing issues raised by those who do not understand, do not support, or actively oppose the eradication effort. Several examples of barriers in vision encountered in disease eradication implementation and methods utilized to address these barriers are described below.

Disease Is Not an Important Problem

Each of the three global eradication programs — smallpox, dracunculiasis (Guinea worm disease, GW), and polio — has faced this issue. Epidemiologic studies (scar surveys for smallpox, lameness surveys for polio, and village searches for GW) were important in defining the magnitude of the problem or, in current terminology, the burden of disease. These studies were especially catalytic when carried out by a respected national figure as occurred in Nigeria, where Professor Nwosu, a Professor of Parasitology and State Minister of Health, was the responsible investigator. Equally important were the studies that documented the developmental costs of the disease, e.g., the cost of GW in terms of school absenteeism and lost agricultural production (Hopkins and Ruiz-Tiben 1991; Hopkins et al. 1995).

Gaining the commitment of decision makers is frequently facilitated through visits to infected villages, where they can see first hand the ravages of disease, e.g., a smallpox infectious disease hospital or a GW-infected village. Key to this process is listening to those affected. The late Becky Johnson, formerly with Africare in Nigeria, reported that village after village identified GW as their number one health priority because of its cost and, more importantly, its repeated year after year toll on agriculture, education, and family life (Withers, pers. comm.). The visit of President Rawlings and President Carter to GW-infected villages in Ghana was the seminal event in increasing Ghanaian awareness and commitment for GW eradication. Involvement of national leaders provides three distinct advantages to a program: (1) it facilitates the elevation of eradication to the cabinet level and opens opportunities for intersectoral involvement and support e.g., military transport of vaccine; (2) it increases access to resources including communications, education, and local government; and (3) it increases information available to the public through radio, television, and the press.

Eradication Is Impossible

Many individuals, both national and international, struggling to improve health with limited resources see eradication as a detour around their own priorities; their path of resistance is that the "task is impossible" and that resources should not be wasted on an impossible task. Others see the political and/or technical barriers as insurmountable. Addressing these concerns requires a systematic approach of information and dialogue on the burden of disease, on the effectiveness of proposed strategies, and long-term costs and benefits.

Eradication Costs Too Much

Eradication is expensive. Even with global support, endemic countries provide a significant proportion of operational costs. Smallpox eradication costs over US$ 300 million, US$ 200 million of which were provided by the infected countries (Fenner et al. 1988). While some of these costs represent salaries already covered in national budgets, field costs not reimbursed through international sources require shifting of budget items or extra-budgetary funding. When health conditions are poor, decision makers take political risks in allocating funds to an initiative where many of those gains will fall to their political successors in government or to the developed world, e.g., the benefits of global poliomyelitis eradication. Dialogue on the economic and political benefits of an eradication initiative is needed to address these concerns. Economic analyses describing the costs and benefits of continuing control activities versus a successful eradication initiative are important in addressing concerns of the ministries of finance and planning.

Eradication Will Divert Resources

This issue involves the concerns of policymakers on the opportunity costs of nonavailability of funds for other developmental priorities, e.g., female education, family planning, water, and sanitation. While certain eradication programs, e.g., GW, recruit resources which would not otherwise be available (donated filter cloth or larvicide for treating infected waters), concerns about the opportunity cost of embarking on an eradication strategy are legitimate and need to be addressed. Closing down health facilities during National Immunization Days (NIDs) illustrates one of these risks. From the perspective of global ethics, more enlightened financing strategies are needed. For GW, where most of the benefits accrue to the infected populations, global funding is a humanitarian act on behalf of the poorest of the poor. In contrast, the financial benefits of polio eradication will fall disproportionately to the developed countries. These countries need to provide funds for global eradication in proportion to their benefits. The decision of the United States Congress to fund support for global poliomyelitis eradication out of domestic health funds is a positive step in global responsibility.

Only if Eradication Strategy Is Integrated as Part of Primary Health Care

This barrier is traditionally cast in the overly debated vertical versus horizontal concerns of the last 20 years, comprehensive versus selective primary health care (PHC) (Walsh and Warren 1979). Behind these debates are three different development strategies: (1) an eradication strategy which identifies and exploits unique opportunities to utilize scientific knowledge to address specific disease problems (e.g., smallpox, GW); (2) an operational strategy allocating resources to those diseases and conditions that carry the greatest burden of disease and are subject to cost-effective affordable interventions (WDR 1993); and (3) a PHC strategy where preeminence is given to decision making and health implementation at the village level as envisioned at Alma-Ata (WHO 1978). Integral to this PHC perspective is the developmental paradigm that those involved, community members, are the ones most competent to identify and prioritize the problems constraining health and the priorities for using resources for development (Hilton, pers. comm.). From this perspective, eradication programs, e.g., polio and measles, with their reliance on external funding, are interpreted as creating dependency and, as such, detrimental to health development.

Rather than dwell on the differences, it is often more productive to focus on areas of overlap and synergy, i.e., what are the potential contributions of eradication programs to the strengthening of disease control and PHC. GW eradication and, to a lesser extent, polio eradication are developing working partnerships with communities. Examples include: (1) the shift in the locus of activity from the health center to the community, (2) the implementers of the main eradication activity, e.g., delivery of polio vaccine by community volunteers or use of GW filters by the householders themselves; and (3) the involvement of the community in assessing effectiveness. This latter point is well illustrated by a GW-infected village in Burkina Faso, where all but two families adopted the use of filters; the following year, the only cases of GW were among those two families (Hopkins, pers. comm.). Success experienced at the grass roots is a powerful incentive for behavioral change in neighboring areas.

BARRIERS IN CONTENT

Traditionally, most health and development issues are discussed and decisions made on technical grounds. The key components of content have been described: "Key to the successful implementation of an eradication strategy is the vision that the problem is important, the strategy exists, the strategy can be successfully implemented, and that the investment is developmentally sound" (Hopkins, pers. comm.). Fulfilling these criteria requires a systematic stepwise plan for implementation including: (1) epidemiologic studies of the disease assessing its burden and dynamics of transmission; (2) research and pilot studies to test acceptability, feasibility, and effectiveness of intervention strategies; and (3) the successful implementation of the strategy at the national and international levels. For example, the national polio experiences in Cuba, Dominican Republic, and Brazil were fundamental in developing the knowledge base on which to launch the program to eliminate poliomyelitis in the Western Hemisphere.

BARRIERS IN CONTEXT

Lack of peace, political stability, or economic stability are barriers to the successful implementation of eradication programs and the achievement of eradication. This is best exemplified by the situation in Sudan, where the civil war has limited the GW program access to the last major endemic area in the world. Ethnic conflict in Ghana has set back that program by at least two years. Polio eradication is encountering similar problems as it moves into Somalia and Central Africa. Political instability and economic chaos, e.g., Nigeria, limit program ability to work effectively and efficiently. Such situations need to be looked at as barriers to overcome rather than insolvable problems. Here, the mind set of the eradication team is critical: how do we implement the essential elements of the eradication strategy within the political and economic realities. Examples of creative approaches to war include J. Grant's, the late Executive Director of UNICEF, brokered days of tranquility in Lebanon and El Salvador for childhood immunization, and President Carter's 4-month cease fire in Sudan for GW. The bottom line is clear: eradication involves politics and will increasingly involve establishing strategic alliances with political decision makers at national and global levels to develop and support eradication activities in troubled areas.

BARRIERS IN PROCESS

The greatest single determinant of successful eradication is that of leadership. Eradication leadership is not a top-down military operation, but the work of an entrepreneur with a vision and a goal (Porter 1995). A review of past and current leaders of eradication initiatives identifies a unique set of characteristics which the author ascribes as "eradication entrepreneurs." Characteristics include global visionary, goal oriented, optimistic, proactive, flexible, charismatic, and, as appropriate, stubborn. The challenge to the entrepreneur is to develop a core team of leaders at national, regional, and international levels to implement a multidisciplinary strategy of advocacy, information-education-communications (IEC), training, operations, surveillance, problem identification and resolution, and the development of strategic alliances.

Team advocacy is well illustrated in the Americas' Poliomyelitis Eradication Programme, where the personal dynamism of Ciro de Quadros, the strong commitment of Regional Director Carlyle G. de Macedo, and the political know-how of Mark Schneider (a former U.S. Under-Secretary of State on detail to the Pan American Health Organization, PAHO) succeeded in getting the issue of poliomyelitis eradication on the agendas of the regional summits of presidents. The PAHO program also provides an excellent example of alliance development, e.g., the coming together of PAHO and Rotary International in polio eradication. Rotary's commitment to polio evolved out of an organizational commitment to health, hunger, and humanity; a desire to celebrate its 75th and later its 100th anniversary; and the advocacy of persuasive Rotarians, including Robert Hingson, a long-term advocate for global immunization using mass campaigns; a physician president; and the technical consultation and advocacy of Albert Sabin (Cook, pers. comm.). While many decision makers saw Rotary as an additional source of funding, PAHO envisioned a Rotary partnership in which individual Rotarians and local Rotary Clubs would contribute through mobilizing political commitment, advocacy and publicity, and in operations at the local level.

Similarly, strategic alliances with industry have been important in implementing the GW program through donations of filter material and larvicide. In terms of broadening the support for eradication, strategic alliances, when identified as beneficial by both parties, are important. Three aspects of establishing these alliances merit emphasis: (1) recognition of the need for strategic alliances with partners outside of the health mainstream with whom common bonds and common goals can be nurtured; (2) a proactive strategy of program advocacy and search for partners; (3) an openness to substantive creative nontraditional inputs that these partners can contribute.

OPERATIONAL BARRIERS

Agency Infighting

Decisions in international health development are made by representatives of national governments, NGOs, international and bilateral development assistance agencies, and increasingly the private sector. Each of these has its own agenda and objectives. Where there are commonalities in agency and eradication program objectives, development of common goals and linkages is relatively easy. Where agency objectives are in conflict, and especially when these conflicts are complicated by interpersonal animosities, agencies may not only withhold support, but may, in fact, actively oppose the implementation of the eradication strategy. Development of inter-agency coordinating committees at global and country levels is an effective mechanism for gaining consensus and resolving problems. At the country level, these meetings should be chaired by a national authority.

Lack of Commitment

Health initiatives in a developing country are traditionally assigned to programs within a Ministry of Health bureaucracy. Seldom, if ever, do these individual programs have the vision, power, and resources needed to gain the national presence required for eradication. Thus, addressing the issue of commitment involves finding a way to elevate eradication to the Minister of Health and, more importantly, to the National Government. In Mali, a languishing GW program was revitalized through the recruitment of the recently retired, politically popular former head of state General Amadou Toumani Toure to head the program. General Toure's advocacy, strengthened by reports from his mother of the burden of GW in her home village, extended beyond Mali to francophone West Africa (Hopkins, pers. comm.). Addressing the barrier of commitment involves finding allies among those at the highest levels of government. At the international level, a bilingual exhibit on GW, which was prepared by CDC and displayed outside the meeting room of the World Health Assembly, was instrumental in bringing the issue to international attention and in the passage of the Guinea worm Eradication Resolution in 1986 (Hopkins, pers. comm.).

Lack of Resources

Four maxims regarding resources are important: (1) eradication programs are expensive; (2) eradication programs always cost more than expected, (3) the cost per case prevented increases incrementally as the number of cases approaches zero, and (4) eradication can be a cost-effective development strategy. Resource needs are both external (technical assistance, vaccines, vehicles) and national (salaries, per diem, publicity). While some of these national costs are in-kind salaries included in the health budget, operational costs not reimbursed from international resources require internal shifting of line items or extra-budgetary funding. Identification and recruitment of resources are a continuing challenge and require four actions: (1) a clear presentation of the issues, (2) a plan that spells out in lay terms the challenge and the progress, (3) a nuclear core of committed funders, and (4) an active search for partners.

Central Control

While there were many scientific reasons for the failure of malaria eradication, a major contributor was the operational philosophy — a centrally controlled top-down implementation of a strategy developed by and approved by WHO Expert Committees (Packard 1997). The malaria program functioned independently of the government health system and lacked the capacity to allow staff to modify procedures to overcome problems identified in the field. Given the existent differences in epidemiology, cultures, and resources, successful disease eradication requires decentralized implementation which allows and promotes a collaborative problem-solving implementation of strategy, provided, however, that issues addressed are critical to the ultimate goal of eradication.

In contrast, the major determinant of the success in smallpox eradication was its ability to evolve its operational strategy as workers in the field found better ways of doing things. Over a 15-year period, the program's operational strategy evolved through three different operational strategies: (1) mass vaccination, (2) mass vaccination with coverage assessment, and (3) surveillance containment. This evolution is better understood in terms of the critical indicators used to measure performance:

- number of vaccinations (1960),
- numbers of vaccinations and percent coverage (1966),
- numbers of cases (1967),
- number of infected villages (1968),
- interval in days between first case and detection (1993),
- interval in days between detection and last case (1994),
- knowledge of reward (1994), and
- number of rash cases detected (1995).

Poliomyelitis surveillance and GW detection and containment are going through similar transformations.

Lack of Community Partnership

Two aspects of community partnerships are important to the success of eradication: cultural factors related to community understanding of the disease, its cause, the appropriateness of its prevention or treatment strategy; and co-opting the public as active responsible partners in the eradication process.

In the early stages of smallpox eradication, smallpox was understood as a visitation of the supernatural (Sopona in Nigeria, Shitla Mata in India, and Allah in Bangladesh). With this perspective, appropriate interventions, if any, related to deity worship. In the GW program there was resistance to "poisoning" the water with larvacide in fear of offending the "sacred crocodile" (Hopkins, pers. comm.). Personal and community preference for the "sweet" taste of GW-infected polluted water provides another example of a cultural barrier. Misunderstanding of an intervention, e.g., tetanus toxoid as a contraceptive, illustrates how the value of an intervention can be compromised by an unexpected perception. While no cultural barrier has been insurmountable, it is important for programs to carry out the applied anthropologic research to identify the cultural barriers and to find culturally acceptable methods of prevention and control.

A personal smallpox experience emphasizes the adaptation of an eradication strategy to the local culture. In Somalia, two methods of isolation were used: camp isolation as taught by the Italians and British, and house isolation as used by WHO in India and Bangladesh. Both methods were failing for cultural reasons: (1) infected adults were not willing to leave their domestic responsibilities, animals, and fields; (2) cultural practices involving visiting the sick, often at 2–3 a.m., compromised the effectiveness of hut isolation. Sleeping on an animal skin in nomadic encampments, I noted a number of thorn circular barriers: one for the cows, one for the goats, and one for the camels. Consulting with local elders, creation of an additional thorn enclosure with a lean-to and latrine for the smallpox case solved the problem. The patient was provided money to ensure care of his or her animals, and a vaccinator guard was recruited and paid to provide food and water and vaccinate visitors. The only failure, thereafter, occurred in a village where it was below the dignity of the male guard to carry water; daily, he sent the female smallpox patient to the well to collect water. The above vignette illustrates the importance of adapting the operational strategy, in this case isolation, in a culturally acceptable manner.

Achievement of eradication also requires the program involvement of the community as active partners, not participants. The concept of partnership reflects respect, ownership, responsibility, and action. Community partnerships vary with the eradication program, e.g., reporting of rash cases in smallpox and serving as vaccinators in containment, administering polio vaccine during polio NIDs and in reporting new cases of paralysis, and using filters and surveillance in GW. Developing this community component involves a sequential bringing on board of national leaders, the health workers who represent the program at the local level, and the community. As reported by Withers (pers. comm.), this transformation occurs when nationals, communities, and health staff realize that their program can make a difference, and that they are responsible for its success or failure.

Two examples presented at this Dahlem Workshop illustrate where community partnerships were essential to program implementation (Gaxotte, pers. comm.). In New Guinea, where the disease Kuru was traced to cannibalism, action by those involved succeeded in eliminating cannibalism and Kuru. Among the Yanomani in the Brazil Amazon, ivermectin was used to treat the inhabitants at the edge of the rainforest. Those treated on the edge carried the new strategy into the interior.

Mismanagement and Corruption

Hiding of disease and misappropriation of funds are potential barriers to eradication at all levels: local, subregional, national, regional, and international. This is illustrated by smallpox experience where three countries actively suppressed the presence of smallpox and blocked international access to their countries. Assessing disease status in countries not associated with WHO (e.g., South Africa, Angola, and Mozambique in the 1970s) also proved to be a barrier to be overcome (Henderson, pers. comm.).

In countries where governmental wages are insufficient to meet daily needs, international programs have been viewed as a source of supplementing income. Such salary supplements are two-edged swords: on one hand, loyalty and a full-time commitment to the initiative are promoted, while on the other, long-term commitment to government is decreased. Modulating this income to a level that is legitimate and justifiable is a significant management challenge.

Mismanagement due to incompetence or corruption is also a risk at international, regional, and national levels. Financial systems with clear guidelines, signed agreements, regular audits, and transparency of accounts are essential elements of eradication initiatives.

CONCLUSION

- Planning and implementing eradication initiatives are complex political, scientific, and logistics challenges.
- Policy formulation depends on actors at community, district, subnational, national, regional, and international levels interacting together to address issues of content, context, and process.
- Success in eradication requires, in addition to science and politics, a dedicated multilevel team bonded together by a common goal of disease eradication.
- Barriers of types described threaten the achievement of the ultimate goal of eradication. Anticipation of barriers, preventive actions to limit their escalation, and a program commitment to barrier identification and resolution are essential to the success of an eradication initiative.

REFERENCES

CDC (Centers for Disease Control and Prevention). 1993. Recommendations of the International Task Force on Disease Eradication. *Morbid. Mortal. Wkly. Rep.* **42 (RR–16)**:1–38.

de Quadros, C.A., B.S. Hersh, and J.M. Olivé et al. 1997. Eradication of wild poliovirus from the Americas: Acute flaccid paralysis surveillance. *J. Infec. Dis.* **175 (Suppl. 1)**:S37–42.

de Quadros, C.A., J.H. Olive, and B.S. Hersh et al. 1996. Measles elimination in the Americas: Evolving strategies. *JAMA* **275**:224–229.

Fenner, F., D.A. Henderson, I. Arita, Z. Jezek, and I.D. Ladnyi. 1988. Smallpox and Its Eradication. Geneva: WHO.

Foster, S.O., D.A. McFarland, and A.M. Johns. 1993. Measles. In: Disease Control Priorities in Developing Countries, ed. D.T. Jamison, W.H. Mosley, A.R. Measham, and J.L. Bordilla, pp. 161–187. Oxford: Oxford Univ. Press.

Hopkins, D.R., and E. Ruiz-Tiben. 1991. Strategies for dracunculiasis eradication. *Bull. WHO* **69**:553–540.

Hopkins, D.R., E. Ruiz-Tiben, T. Ruebush III, A.N. Agle, and P.C. Withers. 1995. Dracunculiasis eradication: March 1995 update. *Am. J. Trop. Med. Hyg.* **52**:14–20.

Packard, R.M. 1997. Malaria dreams: Postwar visions of health and development in the third world. *Med. Anthrop.*, in press.

Porter, R.W. 1995. Knowledge Utilization and the Process of Policy Formulation. Support for Analysis and Research in Africa (SARA). Washington, D.C.: U.S. Agency for Intl. Development, Africa Bureau.

Walsh, J.A., and K.S. Warren. 1979. Selective Primary Health Care. *New Engl. J. Med.* **301**:967–974.

Walt, G., and L. Gilson. 1994. Reforming the health sector in developing countries, the role of policy analysis. *Health Pol. Plan.* **9**:353–370.

WHO. 1978. Alma-Ata 1978, Primary Health Care. Geneva: WHO.

WDR (World Development Report). 1993. Investing in Health. Oxford: Oxford University Press for the World Bank.

12

Advantages and Disadvantages of Concurrent Eradication Programs

S.L. COCHI, R.W. SUTTER, P.M. STREBEL,
A.-R. HENINGBURG, and R.A. KEEGAN
National Immunization Program, Mailstop E–05, Atlanta, GA 30333, U.S.A.

ABSTRACT

Any eradication program requires major human and financial resources and political will to be successful. When concurrent eradication programs are contemplated, the standards for consideration are raised to an even higher level compared with a single eradication program. This chapter describes the advantages and disadvantages of undertaking concurrent eradication programs. Notably, what may be an advantage under one particular set of conditions can become a disadvantage under a different set of conditions. Guidelines are offered for assessing the circumstances under which it may be appropriate to consider conducting concurrent eradication programs. While concurrent eradication programs have certain advantages, there needs to be a globally accepted priority assigned to one particular program over the other(s), as demonstrated by instituting an earlier timetable for eradication to the higher priority disease eradication program.

INTRODUCTION

Conducting an eradication program requires major human and financial resources and political will. Consequently, any decision to undertake concurrent eradication programs cannot be taken lightly. Moreover, to consider the advantages and disadvantages of *concurrent* eradication programs requires categorizing the situation according to one of the following sets of assumptions: (1) either the decision to undertake each eradication program (Program A,B,C, etc.) has already been arrived at based on its own merits — therefore, the objective is to determine whether the advantages of concurrent implementation of the (two or more) eradication programs outweigh any potential disadvantages; or (2) a consensus decision to undertake one of the two (or more) eradication programs (e.g., Program A) has *not* already been made, in which case the objective is to determine whether concurrent implementation with another eradication program offers unique advantages which justify proceeding with both eradication programs. Regardless of which of these two circumstances exists, one must

The Eradication of Infectious Diseases
Edited by W.R. Dowdle and D.R. Hopkins © 1998 John Wiley & Sons Ltd.

consider the main preconditions for undertaking *any* eradication program, because these requirements apply similarly to the decision to undertake eradication programs *concurrently*, and to the significant additional commitment that this decision entails. Yekutiel (1981) formulated a set of preconditions that must be met before an eradication program could be contemplated:

1. There should be a control measure that is completely effective in breaking transmission, simple in application, and relatively inexpensive. If the technical intervention(s) is not as effective, simple, or as inexpensive as was originally believed, then failure of the eradication program can result.

2. The disease should have clinical and epidemiological features facilitating effective case detection and surveillance in the advanced stages of the eradication program. If these factors are lacking, it may be impractical to achieve the goal within acceptable limits of effort and cost.

3. The disease must be of recognized socioeconomic importance, national or international. Unless the burden of disease and economic impact are sufficient to be clearly appreciated and to generate political will and popular support, there is the danger that national financial support for the program will not be forthcoming.

4. There should be a specific reason for eradication, rather than control, of the disease. The demand for sustained, high-quality performance and perseverance in an eradication program runs the danger of failure with consequent significant financial loss. Therefore, a specific reason for pursuing eradication instead of control is needed to justify the calculated risk involved (e.g., the ability to stop vaccination against smallpox following eradication). This special reason may be technical or operational *(and, in our view, should be cost saving)*.

5. There should be adequate financial, administrative, personnel, and health service resources. To the extent possible, the budgetary needs of the anticipated program should be defined *before* deciding to undertake the eradication program, including allowance for special contingencies. A clear commitment of funds from international sources is essential at the start.

6. There should be the necessary socioecological conditions. Consideration should be given in advance of the influence of certain human sociological factors such as major population movements, regular seasonal migrations, dispersal of populations in remote areas, and cultural habits and beliefs that may affect receptivity of population groups to the intervention, on the ultimate success of the eradication program.

Hinman (1966) listed eight criteria that should be considered in proposing a disease as a candidate for eradication:

1. Is eradication technically feasible?
2. Is eradication economically feasible?
3. What is the impact of the disease?
4. Is the eradication proposal economically feasible globally?

6. Is there international appeal for the undertaking?
7. Are there personnel available?
8. Will a vertical program slow down emergence of well-rounded public health programs?
9. What are the economic consequences of failure to eradicate?

Although we will not explore further here the particular criteria, as outlined by Yekutiel (1981) and Hinman (1966), that need to be considered before launching into eradication programs, clearly it is essential that these criteria (and perhaps others) must also be fulfilled in circumstances where concurrent eradication programs are undertaken.

It is relevant here to review the definition of the term "*concurrent.*" There are, in fact, different meanings for this term, which might affect one's perception of the task of defining the advantages and disadvantages of concurrent eradication programs. For example, one set of definitions — acting together, cooperating, in agreement, harmonious — appears to convey that benefits and advantages are automatically derived by conducting eradication programs concurrently, which is clearly not the case. For purposes of this discussion, we have chosen to use the following definition — occurring at the same time, existing together — which is neutral in its tone and carries no implications regarding potential advantages or disadvantages.

ADVANTAGES

More Efficient Resource Allocation

Concurrent eradication programs offer the potential advantage of pooling human and financial resources in a way that allows more efficient and effective utilization of those resources. The advantage to be gained is particularly more likely if the eradication strategies and/or program operational elements for the two diseases are compatible with each other, i.e., they share similar or overlapping characteristics which make it possible for the programs to share human and financial resources. Examples of compatible characteristics include: (a) the intervention can be combined and given together (combining two vaccines such as measles and rubella vaccines, giving oral polio vaccine and vitamin A simultaneously during National Immunization Days, NIDs); (b) combining resources to conduct surveillance; or (c) conducting social mobilization for concurrent eradication programs.

Perhaps the best recent example comes from the experience in the Americas with conducting surveillance for polio and measles in conjunction with ongoing concurrent eradication/elimination programs against both diseases. The Pan American Health Organization (PAHO) has drawn on its experience in achieving the eradication of wild poliovirus from the Americas (de Quadros et al. 1997; Pinheiro et al. 1997) to pursue an initiative to eliminate measles from the Americas by the year 2000 (PAHO 1994; de Quadros et al. 1996). The integrated epidemiological and virological surveillance developed for polio eradication became the foundation for the development of the intensive measles surveillance necessary to support the measles elimination initiative. Conversely, measles surveillance and the measles elimination program have helped to sustain polio (i.e., acute flaccid paralysis) surveillance throughout the period following eradication of wild poliovirus in 1991.

Another example illustrating the potential for advantageously exploiting concurrent eradication programs and efficiently utilizing resources would be to undertake measles and rubella eradication programs together. Surveillance of both of these diseases is based on the detection and case investigation of rash illnesses, and the two vaccines can be combined (although cost is an issue) into a single vaccine injection. While global measles eradication is cost effective (Mark Miller, M.D., Global Program for Vaccines and Immunization, WHO, 1997, pers. comm.), rubella eradication as a single disease eradication initiative does not appear to be cost effective and the rubella disease burden (mortality primarily from fetal death and morbidity due to congenital rubella syndrome, CRS) is not likely to justify the incremental cost from adequate control characterized by the absence of reporting of CRS cases to accomplishment of the eradication of the rubella virus. However, the concurrent eradication of both measles and rubella, using a combination measles–rubella vaccine, is likely to be cost effective and could persuade policymakers to allocate also the additional resources to eradicate rubella should a global measles eradication goal be adopted in the next few years.

Broader Cooperation and Enhanced Partnership

Concurrent eradication programs offer the opportunity to seek and obtain a broader partnership among international and bilateral organizations, agencies, and governments. This broader partnership may be in the common interest and lead to creation of a larger coalition to eradicate both diseases. The coalition may be motivated because the concurrent eradication programs have compatible strategies and objectives, or because of complementarity (but not incompatibility) between each eradication program's strategies and objectives such that all of the coalition partners perceive advantages in joining forces together.

In the Americas, national initiatives for the control or elimination of measles emerged from the successful organization of NIDs for polio eradication (Olivé et al. 1997). Measles elimination in these countries and in the region as a whole built upon the success of polio eradication in developing a multisectoral coalition to generate the needed financial resources, and in generating intense community and private sector involvement.

In an increasing number of countries, polio NIDs have been combined with the concurrent mass administration of vitamin A to the target population of children age years, a program which, in some countries, has led to the virtual elimination of vitamin A deficiency (Bloem and Gorstein 1995; Loevinsohn et al. 1997; Tangermann et al. 1997). Such activities have fostered collaborations between the polio eradication program and organizations and individuals involved in the prevention of micronutrient deficiency diseases.

There is as yet unrealized potential for cooperation in the context of the activities of the concurrent dracunculiasis and polio eradication programs in Africa (Hopkins and Ruiz-Tiben 1991) that could contribute positively to both programs, as well as potentially lead to more efficient use of existing resources. Such cooperation might possibly occur in one of at least two forms: (1) joint activities in difficult areas such as occurred on a limited basis in southern Sudan during the 4-month period of the "Guinea Worm Cease-Fire" in 1995 (WHO 1996); and (2) joint sharing of resources, expertise, and cooperation in disease surveillance for Guinea worm and polio. The latter issue has just recently become the subject of discussion and has yet to result in a consensus. The differences in the epidemiology, geographic distribution, and control measures of these two diseases are important factors in determining whether there are overlapping characteristics and surveillance functions that are amenable to sharing resources to achieve enhanced surveillance of these diseases. Whereas dracunculiasis tends to occur in remote, sparsely populated, rural villages unserved or minimally served by the health system, such settings are not where poliovirus circulation is likely to persist; rather, densely populated urban or peri-urban areas are more favorable conditions for the continued circulation of poliovirus and maintenance of a reservoir. Whereas, dracunculiasis surveillance is predominantly village- and community-based and requires the identification, treatment, and containment of every affected person (who is subject to becoming reinfected), the primary goal of polio surveillance is to identify infected districts in need of appropriate actions (finding every case is not an absolute requirement), and surveillance is predominantly health facility-based with paralytic cases serving as sentinel events to identify an infected population.

Synergy of Political Commitment and Popular Support

Concurrent eradication programs have the potential to enhance the mobilization of political support, and capture greater public attention and popular support. An example of this phenomenon is the situation that existed in Cuba and the English-speaking Caribbean countries in 1985 and thereafter, when PAHO began the campaign to eradicate poliomyelitis from the Americas. Although these countries were already free of polio, they participated in the polio eradication initiative while becoming the first countries in the Americas (Cuba in 1987, English-speaking Caribbean in 1991) to field test and implement the PAHO measles elimination strategies that were still under development during that period (de Quadros et al. 1996). Hence, these countries concurrently participated in polio eradication and set the pace on measles for other countries in the Americas while addressing a disease that, within their own countries, was higher on their list of health priorities than polio. Programs that combine eradication of polio or measles with elimination of vitamin A deficiency disease, or concurrent eradication of measles and rubella using a combination vaccine, represent other examples. The program to eradicate smallpox and control measles in West and Central Africa in the late 1960s to early 1970s is another example of synergistic collaboration — in that program, the United States' interest in smallpox eradication was joined with the African countries' greater interest in controlling measles.

DISADVANTAGES

Competition for Resources

Earlier in this chapter we pointed out that conducting an eradication program requires major human and financial resources. Given this reality, there is substantial danger of failure in conducting concurrent eradication programs without having adequate financial, administrative, personnel, and health services resources available or committed to carry out *each* eradication program before deciding to undertake these programs concurrently. A clear commitment of significant funds from international sources for each program is essential before any serious consideration is possible. In the absence of adherence to these criteria, proceeding with concurrent eradication efforts can have a profound negative impact on one or both programs. A lack of a clear commitment of substantial resources for accelerated neonatal tetanus prevention was one of the factors contributing to the failure to achieve the goal of elimination by the year 1995, while concurrent efforts in the polio eradication program, which have had increasingly substantial funding commitments, have continued to demonstrate dramatic progress.

Farid (1980) contends that the final blow dealt, beginning in the mid-1960s, to the failed malaria eradication program was to slash the malaria eradication budget and transform the single purpose malaria surveillance program staff into multipurpose health workers to meet the new demands of the new internationally assisted programs in smallpox eradication, family planning, and development of basic health services. He claimed that "the global smallpox campaign . . . . took full advantage of the facilities existing in the national malaria eradication services and was a factor in accelerating their dismantling."

Lack of Cooperation and Coordination

An unintended, but disastrous, side effect of concurrent eradication programs could be a deterioration or complete breakdown in cooperation and coordination among the partners involved in these programs, especially if not all partners are involved in both (all) programs. One potential scenario is that if the programs lack compatible strategies and objectives, the incentive to cooperate and coordinate activities may be lost. In this scenario, each eradication program would develop its own infrastructure and verticality, and interagency coordination would be compromised. Such circumstances might also increase the likelihood of detracting from routine public health programs.

Divided or Diluted Political Commitment and Popular Support

Concurrent eradication programs run the risk of dividing or diluting enthusiasm and political support between the individual eradication programs and, hence, lessening the likelihood of success of either program. With the divided political commitment may come a lack of focus on what is truly needed by each eradication program to achieve adequate political commitment and popular support both nationally and at the community level.

Eradication of a causative agent (i.e., virus, bacteria, parasite) is resource-intensive and requires substantial efforts over a limited period, not only in terms of securing the incremental funding needed to progress from control to eradication, but also in terms of allocating scarce human resources. Thus, a decision to adopt a new eradication target must be made only after careful deliberation regarding all related issues; otherwise, competition among the disease eradication targets could result, which would dramatically increase the likelihood of failure of at least one of these initiatives. A failure of any one of these initiatives could seriously jeopardize other eradication initiatives in the future by affecting funding decisions (both from external donors and within countries) for these initiatives as well.

CONCLUSIONS

An eradication program requires major human and financial resources and political will to be successful. Multiple concurrent eradication programs test the limits of this principle even further than does a single eradication program. Therefore, concurrent eradication programs may be appropriate and are most likely to be successful only if, in general, the following special set of circumstances can be fulfilled:

1. The technical feasibility of each eradication program is reasonably assured because the intervention is effective, simple in application, and relatively inexpensive, and the strategies for achieving eradication have been successfully tested in a large geographic area.
2. Each of the diseases under consideration is of recognized public health importance and there is broad international appeal for undertaking their eradication.
3. Together, the concurrent programs engender greater financial and human resource commitments and political will in a manner that suggests, on economic grounds, the feasibility of success.
4. The interventions and strategies are compatible with each other in the implementation phase, thus optimizing efficient use of resources, cooperation, and coordination among national governments and the partner organizations involved.
5. A global consensus exists that concurrent, as opposed to sequential, eradication efforts should be undertaken for these diseases, despite the additional risks, in order to speed the delivery of health benefits to the world's population.

Of note, the lists of advantages and disadvantages regarding concurrent eradication programs that have been outlined herein form mirror images of one another. What may be an advantage under one particular set of conditions can become a disadvantage under a different set of conditions. We conclude that whether concurrent eradication programs are, on balance, advantageous or disadvantageous compared with undertaking separate, sequential, single disease eradication programs depends entirely on: (a) the nature and characteristics of the particular diseases and programs themselves; and (b) the degree to which cooperation, coordination, political commitment, and popular support can be enhanced. We have offered some guidelines for determining when it may be appropriate to consider undertaking eradication programs concurrently. While concurrent eradication programs have certain advantages, there needs to be a globally accepted priority assigned to one particular program over the other(s), as demonstrated by instituting an earlier timetable for eradication to the higher priority disease eradication program.

REFERENCES

Bloem, M.W., and J. Gorstein. 1995. Viet Nam: Xerophthalmia free. 1994 National vitamin A deficiency and protein-energy malnutrition prevalence survey. Helen Keller International, consultancy report, March 5–17, 1995.

de Quadros, C.A., B.S. Hersh, J.M. Olivé, J.K. Andrus, C.M. da Silveira, and P.A. Carrasco. 1997. Eradication of wild poliovirus from the Americas: Acute flaccid paralysis surveillance, 1988–1995. *J. Infec. Dis.* **175 (Suppl 1)**:S37–42.

de Quadros, C.A., J.M. Olivé, B.S. Hersh, M.A. Strassburg, D.A. Henderson, D. Brandling-Bennett, and G.A.O. Alleyne. 1996. Measles elimination in the Americas: Evolving strategies. *JAMA* **275**:224–229.

Farid, M.A. 1980. The malaria program — From euphoria to anarchy. *World Hlth. For.* **1**:8–33.

Hinman, E.H. 1966. World Eradication of Infectious Diseases. Springfield: C.C. Thomas.

Hopkins, D.R., and E. Ruiz-Tiben. 1991. Strategies for dracunculiasis eradication. *Bull. WHO* **69**:533–540.

Loevinsohn, B.P., R.W. Sutter, and M.O. Costales. 1997. Using cost-effectiveness analysis to evaluate targeting strategies: The case of vitamin A supplementation. *Health Pol. Plan.* **12**:29–37.

Olivé, J.M., J.B. Risi, and C.A. de Quadros. 1997. National immunization days: Experience in the Americas. *J. Infec. Dis.* **175 (Suppl 1)**:S189–193.

PAHO (Pan American Health Organization). 1994. Measles elimination by the year 2000. *EPI Newsl.* **14(No. 5)**:1–2.

Pinheiro, F.P., O.M. Kew, M.H. Hatch, C.M. da Silveira, and C.A. de Quadros. 1997. Eradication of wild poliovirus from the Americas: Wild poliovirus surveillance — Laboratory issues. *J. Infec. Dis.* **175 (Suppl. 1)**:S43–49.

Tangermann, R.H., M. Costales, and J. Flavier. 1997. Poliomyelitis eradication and its impact on primary health care in the Philippines. *J. Infec. Dis.* **175 (Suppl. 1)**:S272–276.

WHO (World Health Organization). 1996. Dracunculiasis: Global surveillance summary, 1995. *Wkly. Epidemiol. Rec.* **71**:141–148.

Yekutiel, P. 1981. Lessons from the big eradication campaigns. *World Hlth. For.* **2**:465–490.

13

Designing Eradication Programs to Strengthen Primary Health Care

C.E. TAYLOR[1] and R.J. WALDMAN[2]

[1]Dept. of International Health, School of Hygiene and Public Health,
Johns Hopkins University, Baltimore, MD 21205, U.S.A.
[2]BASICS, Suite 300, Arlington, VA 22209, U.S.A.

INTRODUCTION

Over the past few decades, great progress has been made in learning how to implement both eradication programs and primary health care. It is now possible to focus on bringing the two together. Country officials and donors alike are saying that integration is needed. Two-way benefits are possible because while eradication programs depend greatly on health infrastructure, they also can help build health systems if done right. Better understanding of the dynamics of systematic integration will help in making future interactions synergistic. Yet before progress can be realized, we will need to face frankly past problems in relationships.

BACKGROUND

A significant shift has occurred in the organization of eradication programs. Early programs, such as for malaria in the 1950s and 1960s, were organized as quasi-military campaigns with narrowly focused short-term objectives, strong hierarchical control, meticulous rigor in details of implementation, a limited range of technical interventions, little field flexibility, and more concern about accommodating uncertainties of mosquito ecology than human social and cultural constraints. People were not consulted and their compliance was taken for granted. Technical experts and government officials were in control.

A significant long-term contribution of malaria eradication efforts, however, was to demonstrate in diverse situations that health workers could reach all clusters of homes, however remote, with a scientifically based intervention. For the first time, a health service was provided for everyone in a poor country, thus demonstrating that equity was possible. Since that time, each new eradication program has stimulated

The Eradication of Infectious Diseases
Edited by W.R. Dowdle and D.R. Hopkins © 1998 John Wiley & Sons Ltd.

incremental learning about how health programs can adjust to the needs and concerns of local people, flexibly adapt to political and social realities, and integrate with local services.

In the past half century much has also been learned about primary health care. Most countries now have some health care infrastructure and therefore integration seems more feasible. Primary health care is a rather new concept that bridges the traditional gap separating public health from curative medicine. The concept is rather new; the first practical demonstration of primary health care in a developing country was the Ding Xian experiment in China in the 1930s. Many projects around the world have now shown that simplified curative and preventive interventions can be provided to families in community-based activities that reach total populations, including the poor and most needy. Behavior change and simple but effective interventions introduced by community workers produce significant and sustainable impact. Community empowerment approaches can work under any political, social, or economic system. With varying combinations of public funding and community financing, primary health care can now be promoted in ways that produce self-reliance, not dependency.

The 1978 Alma-Ata World Conference on Primary Health Care stimulated a worldwide movement to build health systems in developing countries. Problems continue, however, in learning how community-based programs can go to scale. In the past decade and a half, as earlier health development has been reversed by economic adjustment policies, there have been severe cutbacks in funding for health services within countries and internationally. Eradication programs also face increasing competition in access to sharply limited resources.

THE ECONOMICS OF INTEGRATION

In considering how costs for eradication should be allocated, it seems reasonable that when a disease selected for global eradication does not have high priority in a particular country, then most costs should be provided from external sources. This would represent a shift from the experience with polio eradication in the Americas, where 80% of costs were borne by host countries. Polio would normally have low priority in most of Africa while measles would have high priority; Guinea worm disease (dracumculiasis) would also have high priority in areas where it occurs. Even if external costs are completely covered, eradication activities make great demands on health systems and many routine activities are inevitably neglected. These opportunity costs also should be covered by clearly defined, compensating benefits when the disease has low priority locally.

Going beyond immediate costs, it is worth noting that global eradication cannot proceed without the cooperation of the countries where endemic infections will remain as global eradication proceeds in most of the world. At the same time the health needs of these countries are increasingly being ignored by donors who are cutting back support worldwide (Evans 1995; WHO 1995; UN Children's Fund 1995). It seems worth considering that donors might be more inclined to provide sustainable support for health systems if the two-way linkages between eradication and primary health care could be more clearly defined. For instance, National Immunization Days (NIDs) are the main hope for achieving polio eradication in Africa. Evidence from West Africa indicates that in countries where there is a very weak health infrastructure, recent NIDs achieved about half the coverage with oral polio vaccine that was achieved in countries where the UNICEF Bamako Initiative provided minimum health coverage in villages (pers. comm., R. Knippenberg, West Africa regional office of UNICEF, February, 1997). Such a service provides credibility that encourages participation in NIDs since in most places there is high priority demand for simple drugs. Similarly, donors might be more attracted to primary health care programs if these had specific disease control targets which, when reached, would represent a potential jumping-off point for eradication programs. The World Health Assembly resolution endorsing polio eradication, for example, explicitly "encourages Member States which have not yet attained a 70% coverage rate to accelerate their efforts so as to surpass this level . . . through means which also improve and sustain the coverage for the other vaccine. . . . This improvement of low vaccination coverage is a responsibility of all primary health care programs."

It also seems possible that eradication programs can be a catalyst for specific health activities. For example, NIDs could be used for supplementary programs, such as giving all of the EPI vaccines and Vitamin A. Costs would necessarily increase, and a provision should be made so that the added services continue after NIDs for eradication are no longer needed. It would be more useful, however, to develop management and logistics services during eradication such that sustainable improvement is achieved to avoid, as has happened in the past, the collapse of whole systems after outside support is terminated. It is true that integration adds to the cost of achieving the single objective of eradication; however, when the synergistic benefits of meeting multiple objectives are brought together, there are remarkable economies achieved in overall costs. Most important, benefits can be sustained in the whole health system.[1]

DIFFICULTIES IN INTEGRATING ERADICATION PROGRAMS AND PRIMARY HEALTH CARE

Recent multicountry evaluations have made it abundantly clear that eradication programs are most effectively and efficiently implemented where there is an existing

---

[1] In some countries, where the health system has been paralyzed or destroyed by war, civil strife, or other conditions incompatible with routine public health activities, narrowly targeted programs such as polio eradication cannot be and should not be expected to achieve the impossible. In such situations, these programs can offer important health benefits that would not otherwise be available to the population.

health infrastructure (PAHO 1995; Taylor et al. 1996). Eradication programs logically grow out of progressive improvements in health systems. In the normal evolution of primary health care, the introduction of an effective scientific intervention may reach a point where control or elimination of a specific disease in particular regions of the world is possible. When a decision is made to proceed with an eradication effort there may be a tendency to make it a vertical rather than an integrated program. Past experience has shown that major intrinsic difficulties need to be understood for mutually synergistic implementation.

A Pan American Health Organization (PAHO) evaluation in six countries in the Americas showed that there were three times more positive comments about the impact of polio eradication on health services than negative comments (PAHO 1995). From the smallpox experience, the PAHO program learned the importance of conducting eradication as part of health services. Positive impact on health services was noted, especially in promoting social mobilization, management, intersectoral cooperation, and a culture of prevention. However, there were also clearly defined negative effects which included: excessive pressures from targeting, population fatigue from single purpose visits to homes, diversion of effort from other health programs, and top-down "paternalistic" attitudes in setting priorities. A firm conclusion was that achieving this balance of more positive than negative effects depended on the fact that the countries studied already had a well-established health infrastructure and that these findings should not be directly extrapolated to countries without equivalent health systems.

Another systematic study of the impact of mass immunization programs was an evaluation of UNICEF's Universal Child Immunization (UCI) programs with vaccines against six diseases (Taylor et al. 1996). This study was done in six countries in Africa and Asia, where health conditions tended to be much worse than in the Americas and with less effective coverage by health services. The goal of 80% coverage of the world's children by 1990 was achieved by UCI through greatly increased outreach to remote and neglected areas. However, these targeted immunization programs tended not to be uniformly sustainable in the poorest countries with weak infrastructure. Global goals had been implemented aggressively, overriding local priorities. Where local capacity was inadequate, parallel structures for support, logistics, and administration had been set up which often collapsed when external funding was withdrawn. Complaints were common about imposition of top-down social mobilization.

The practical conclusion is that future mass programs need to distinguish between countries that do and do not have adequate health infrastructure and that eradication programs should take the time to strengthen or build health systems. Although it is not always the case, some eradication programs, such as the polio eradication initiative, have not focused on countries with weak health infrastructure until late in the effort, because it is natural to concentrate first on countries where results can be achieved rapidly. Then international pressure builds up with growing impatience to meet artificial and over-optimistic deadlines. Poor countries and poor areas of all countries are eventually targeted and, by then, there is little willingness to strengthen health systems in the places that need help most. Programs revert to imposing a top-down hierarchy as outsiders take control to meet deadlines and past lessons about building health systems are ignored.

Eradication programs can do better. Flexibility in timing should be built into planning. The countries that need health system strengthening should not be left to the last and subjected to international pressure when they are holding up the global goal. The usual publicity given to international comparisons makes leaders feel so embarrassed in front of their national neighbors that they feel they must support the global goal, even though the disease being eradicated may be a minor problem as compared with diseases killing many thousands of their own children. These leaders are then pressured to divert large proportions of their domestic resources and attention to global eradication. It is the ethical responsibility of donor countries to realize that global goals cannot succeed without the cooperation of the poorest countries and that they are obligated, especially in situations of greatest need, to pay most attention to improving health infrastructure (Taylor et al. 1997).

PRACTICAL STEPS IN THE PROCESS OF STRENGTHENING PRIMARY HEALTH CARE INFRASTRUCTURE DURING ERADICATION PROGRAMS

The following practical procedures may help efforts to integrate services, even where great differences are found in country health systems. It must be realized, however, there are no universal solutions or silver bullets. Instead an effort must be made to apply what seems to be a universal process to help find appropriate local solutions.

1. Past polarization between proponents of primary health care and those of eradication programs represents an exaggerated example of continuing controversies between vertical and horizontal programs. It is time to admit that this is a false polarization which has become unnecessarily emotional and irrational. It is false because both top-down and bottom-up approaches are needed but for different functions.

2. To resolve the polarization, a straightforward method is to do a *functional analysis* to distinguish top-down functions from those that should be bottom-up. In each situation, different capabilities among partners require that the functional analysis be adapted to work out the role reallocation appropriate to that area. In many countries around the world rapid decentralization makes it essential to reallocate roles between central and peripheral partners. Three levels are outlined in Table 14.1 (see Cochi et al., this volume) to help define the roles of partners at the central/provincial level, district level, and community or most peripheral administrative unit level.

3. A very positive trend in health care programming is that greater attention is being paid to promoting equity. One of the positive arguments for eradication programs is that they show that equity is possible because they reach everyone.

However, a serious problem in recent country efforts to decentralize has been that economic adjustment policies have greatly reduced the public funds available to health services. As decentralization filters money and authority downward in the hierarchy, the process usually stops at the district level. This often makes previous inequity worse because the most efficient and repressive discrimination is often at this level. Conditions for the poor deteriorate as local elites use decentralization to strengthen their position and reinforce ancient patterns of exploitation. A rationalized process of functional analysis has the great benefit that it can be designed to promote both efficiency and equity by setting standards that district and community leaders have to meet.

4. The social mobilization that makes such activities as NIDs possible benefits from diverse traditions of community organization and action. Experience around the world shows that community-based projects can build capacity and empower local people to solve their own problems under any political, social, or economic system. Thousands of local projects have been successful under extremely diverse conditions, and they can be found in almost every country.

5. A major problem has been that successful community-based projects have not typically done well in "going to scale" or rapid expansion. Every community's situation and local solutions tend to be different. We are learning, however, to apply a universal process to find the solutions that are most appropriate locally. A small UNICEF monograph prepared for the World Summit on Social Development in Copenhagen describes such a SCALE–SEED process (Taylor-Ide and Taylor 1995).

   SCALE refers to three stages of scaling up:
   (a) SCALE One (Selecting Communities As Learning Examples) starts the process by mobilizing local projects in each region that have been most successful in community empowerment;
   (b) A SCALE-Squared Center (Self-help Center for Action Learning and Experimentation) is developed in each region by building capacity for participatory education and research in selected SCALE One projects;
   (c) A SCALE-Cubed Process (Sustainable Collaboration for Adaptive Learning and Extension) then organizes the SCALE-Squared Centers into a network for regional expansion.

   SEED stands for Self-Evaluation with Essential Data. At each level, capacity for problem-solving is developed to balance specific contributions in a three-way partnership of communities, officials, and experts. The officials may come from government or nongovernment organizations, religion, business, or special agencies. Experts from academic and research organizations help merge local wisdom with international scientific expertise. Intensive dialogue defines issues, gathers data with involvement of community members, analyzes it locally, and then uses the findings for joint packaging of services to address global and local priorities. The regional SCALE-Squared Centers adapt a simplified social mobilization and action package for extension to all communities in the region.

6. A key activity in integrating eradication and health systems is to develop a methodology for balancing global and local priorities. SCALE-SEED and functional analysis methods provide a framework for such balancing of priorities. For instance, a systematic process is needed to promote social mobilization for NIDs. Where health systems are well-organized, cooperative activities can build on trust from earlier intersectoral and voluntary action; however, a common problem is that after a few rounds of NIDs, spontaneous enthusiasm tends to diminish. To achieve sustainability, an organizational base is needed so local workers can receive a continuing stimulus of recognition and publicity. SCALE-SEED can provide a community-based framework for such action. Where there is no existing health infrastructure the need for this kind of organization to stimulate self-reliant action is even more important.

FUNCTIONAL ANALYSIS TO INTEGRATE ERADICATION AND PRIMARY HEALTH CARE OBJECTIVES

To help integrate eradication and primary health care, a framework was delineated by Cochi et al. during this workshop (see Table 14.3, this volume) to illustrate possible parameters that should be considered when doing a functional analysis. In this balancing of top-down and bottom-up approaches, each row in the matrix describes a function that is distributed to reallocate roles at three levels: central/provincial, district, and community. The functions in the rows of the matrix are not sequential steps, and they can be combined, done in different order, or perhaps skipped entirely.

Part 1: Program Design, Planning, and Information System

1. The process usually begins with a decision by national leaders to participate in an international eradication effort. As was done in the 1988 World Health Assembly resolution, which initiated the global polio eradication program, it is important for a commitment to be made from the beginning that the eradication effort will strengthen primary health care infrastructure. The initiative for this essentially top-down decision will primarily come from national leaders.

2. Joint planning committees should be set up to go beyond interagency coordination among donors and to start relationships that form long-term partnerships with representatives of communities, officials, and experts. At the central level, the joint planning committee has primary responsibility for the functional analysis. The reallocation of roles should be flexible since the availability of personnel will differ in various parts of the country. As SCALE One projects are upgraded to SCALE-Squared Centers they can provide a framework for organizing district level partnership teams. As a network of SCALE-Squared

Centers develops, each can bring together local partnerships of community members, officials, and experts. At each level it is essential to include representatives of the poor and others previously left out of decision making, especially women.

3. Developing an equity framework and establishing firm standards for reaching groups in greatest need is primarily a top-down function. Eradication programs can take the lead in showing that equity is possible. This difficult but essential responsibility cannot simply be left to local decision makers. Local elites are adept at using new benefits to strengthen their position, and they often manipulate development programs to increase exploitation and discrimination. Decentralization may result in power being delegated to the district level, where those in power consolidate control and corruption more efficiently than people at the central level can readily do. For equity to reach those in greatest need, strong performance standards should be set at the national level so that district hierarchies and community elites have to ensure that benefits reach the poorest groups, especially women and children.

4. A surveillance and monitoring framework must be set up at the central level but its application should be at the local and district levels. A basic epidemiologic principle is that in controlling disease in a population, the first step is to identify the groups that have the problem and then concentrate control measures among them. Inefficiencies in setting up surveillance for single diseases can be compensated for by packaging indicators for several priority problems. A more efficient long-term process is to develop surveillance for equity (Taylor 1992). Many problems are concentrated in population groups that are poor and neglected, and close monitoring of the most needy families may be an efficient way of following indicators for several locally important diseases. Surveillance has two components: reporting and response. The reporting should come from the local level, but the response is often best coordinated from the district level where epidemiological expertise is maintained.

5. Priority setting is a central focus of effective planning, and a delicate balance is needed between central and community concerns. Eradication has priority centrally, but probably not for the community. To involve communities, "entry points" are used to emphasize relationships between successful global activities and those activities in demand locally, in an effort to create an awareness that will lead the community to accept a global priority.

6. Social mobilization stimulates action at all levels. At the central level this may be a function that appeals to leaders. Giving polio vaccine has public appeal and it is good politics to be shown on television giving a dose to an obviously needy child or even to a beautiful and happy child. At the district level, intersectoral collaboration can then be promoted in the name of national leaders. From the beginning social mobilization should be planned to be

sustainable rather than as a transitory event. Partnerships can be formed in specific mass activities that move on to address packages of other local priorities involving officials from government, nongovernment organizations, religion, business, media, and entertainment. NIDs can be used to build capacity, self-confidence, and a culture of prevention.

7. Financing is where planning must eventually focus in order to assure sustainability. For many, but not all, diseases that are the target of eradication programs, donor countries will usually receive the greatest benefits from the promotion of global eradication. For instance, it is estimated that the U.S. will save US$ 230 million in vaccine costs each year when polio immunizations are no longer needed. Donors should therefore share these benefits with the poorest countries whose cooperation is needed to achieve eradication.

Part 2: Implementation

1. Areas where health systems are weak pose the greatest challenge to integration of eradication activities with the provision of broader health services. Wherever possible, the scaling-up process (described above) should take advantage of common features shared by different programs. For example, polio eradication activities could be combined with the control of other vaccine-preventable diseases, such as measles, and the delivery of micronutrient supplements to the same target population where health officials feel that these programs are of high priority. Similarly, training, drug procurement and distribution, monitoring, and other essential elements of public health programs can be combined for diarrheal disease control, the control of acute respiratory infections, malaria control, and so forth. Combining individual programs by taking advantage of their common elements can result in enormous economies of scale and effort. However, the pressure of deadlines in eradication programs often mitigates against taking the time and money to build local systems beyond what is required for the eradication program (Siddiqui 1995). The process of integrating eradication efforts into a sustainable health care infrastructure would require different, and slower, timetables than the ones usually offered by proponents of eradication.

2. Training is a central function in scaling up. At the central level the priority is to train trainers. At the district level an extension process is needed to train supervisory and support staff as well as technical workers, especially to work in SCALE-Squared Centers. At the local level these centers then train local leaders, community health workers, and family members by intensive use of learning from people actually doing the practical work involved. Throughout, much support is needed from available media and distance learning. The kind of practical training that is typically required for an eradication program can now be made part of a more comprehensive and sustainable effort.

3. Supervision is a parallel activity that makes training sustainable and useful. The key concept is that supervision should be supportive, going much beyond the punitive rigidity typical of many hierarchies. At the central level the framework for, and training of, supervisors needs to be managed carefully to ensure that eradication goals are met. At the district level the concept of supportive supervision must be integrated with continuing education. At the community level the challenge is to promote community supervision and feedback. Such feedback should also contribute to better performance by professionals and officials.

4. Effective promotion of social mobilization for an eradication effort requires better understanding of cultural constraints and facilitating factors. Scientific knowledge merged with traditional wisdom can be built into community-based, self-reliant action. The choice of what scientific knowledge is relevant should come not only from technical experts but also should include social scientists.

5. Any effective field program depends on communication channels that work and wheels, whether bicycles or four-wheel drive vehicles. The logistics to make equipment, supplies, and means of reporting and transmitting messages effective is part of good management. These are activities that eradication programs have tended to do exceptionally well but their improvements have tended not to be sustainable because long-term maintenance, replacement, and support was not provided for.

6. A framework for quality assurance and meeting performance standards can be facilitated by modern methods of *total quality assurance* simplified for field implementation. At the district or SCALE-squared level there is special need for a team that uses performance indicators and rapid feedback to identify problems early and that mobilizes a continuing search for appropriate corrective measures as programs go to scale. Performance standards need to be balanced with the equally important need for flexibility in adapting to local realities. All activities must be designed to build local capacity.

7. Evaluation follows naturally in the cyclic process of moving from planning to implementation to replanning and incrementally improving services. At the central level, evaluation is best done periodically with external expertise to validate and guide progress. This is especially needed to keep a focus on eradication objectives. At the district level there is more need for continuing monitoring and internal evaluation for flexible adaptation of control measures. It is at the community level that reorientation for local capacity building is most needed through promoting the SEED process. Recent experience in community-based data gathering, causal analysis, and participatory research shows that communities often have more capacity for getting and using reliable information than most professionals had thought. When people participate they believe and use the data, and this leads directly to behavior change and new community norms.

SUMMARY

The process outlined above may seem complex and impractical, especially in contrast to the apparent simplicity of a single purpose, precisely defined goal of eradicating a specific pathogen. However, most of the steps in the functional analysis are important in any eradication program where they may seem sharply focused and therefore more cost-effective. It is also easier to raise money for an objective that is as easily understood as eradication. It may also be claimed that comprehensive health services can be developed best by starting with vertical programs that can be integrated later. The reality is, however, that abundant experience shows that trying to integrate two or more well-established vertical programs is an especially slow and difficult process, partly because vertically oriented staff vigorously resist any loss of their carefully developed identity and mystique. Rather than having to develop each of the above functions in a separate vertical program, we believe it is more efficient to organize sustainable infrastructure for all programs. An emerging challenge is to move on to comprehensive integration of all aspects of social development and ecological preservation through community-based capacity building.

REFERENCES

Evans, I. 1995. SAPping maternal health. *Lancet* **346**:1046. [Note: SAP stands for Structual Adjustment Programs.]

PAHO. 1995 (March). The Impact of the Expanded Programme on Immunization and the Polio Eradication Initiative on Health Systems in the Americas, Final Report of the Taylor Commission. Washington, D.C.: Pan American Health Organization.

Siddiqui, J. 1995. World Health and World Politics. Case Study (Part III): The Malaria Eradication Program, pp. 123–192. Columbia, SC: Univ. of South Carolina Press.

Taylor, C. 1992. Surveillance for equity in primary health care: Policy implications from international experience. *Intl. J. Epidemiol.* **21**:1043–l049.

Taylor, C., F. Cutts, and M.E. Taylor. 1997. Ethical dilemmas in current planning for polio eradication. *Am. J. Pub. Hlth.* **87(6)**:922–925.

Taylor, M.E., F.M. LaForce, R.N. Basu, F. Cutts, P. Ndumbe, and R. Steinglass. 1996. Sustainability of achievements: Lessons learned from universal child immunization. Report of a steering committee. New York: United Nations Children's Fund.

Taylor-Ide, D., and C. Taylor. 1995. Community-Based Sustainable Human Development — Going to Scale with Self-Reliant Social Development. New York: UNICEF Environment Section.

UN Children's Fund. 1995. Health Strategy for UNICEF. New York: United Nations Children's Fund.

WHO. 1995. Bridging the Gaps. Geneva: WHO.

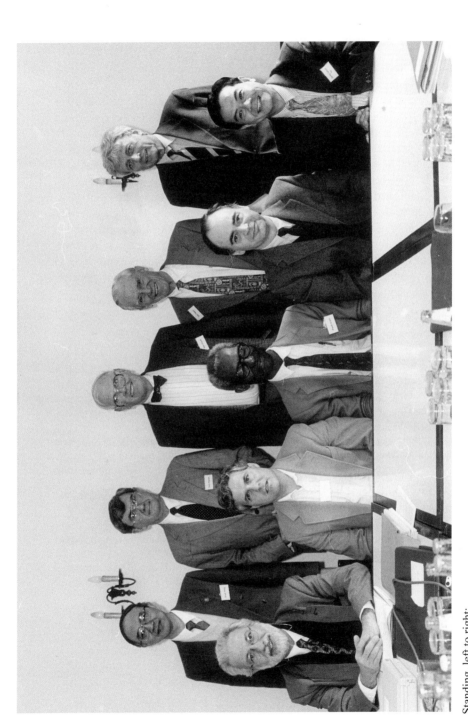

Standing, left to right:
Wang Ke-an, Herb Pigman, Stan Foster, Carl Taylor, Sieghart Dittmann
Seated, left to right:
Ciro de Quadros, Steve Cochi, Frank Grant, Jean-Marc Olivé, Jimmy Galvez Tan

14

Group Report: What Are the Societal and Political Criteria for Disease Eradication?

S.L. COCHI, Rapporteur

C.A. DE QUADROS, S. DITTMANN, S.O. FOSTER,
J.Z. GALVEZ TAN, F.C. GRANT, J.-M. OLIVÉ,
H.A. PIGMAN, C.E. TAYLOR, WANG K.

INTRODUCTION

One of the keys to the success of any public health initiative is the level of societal and political commitment that such initiative is accorded. This is particularly true for eradication initiatives, which need unambiguous and unwavering commitment from start to finish. For infectious diseases of global distribution, it is necessary to be able to persuade all affected countries to implement eradication interventions and maintain them within a defined period. The success of any country in sustaining elimination of the disease is contingent on the success of every country in doing so. It is only through this cumulative success that the entire world can reap the long-term benefits of global eradication of the disease. Even for those infectious diseases which have a limited geographical distribution, successful elimination by one country is closely tied to the success of its neighbors. Improving our understanding of the societal and political conditions that influence eradication programs is fundamental to ensuring the ultimate success of disease eradication.

WHAT ARE THE LESSONS LEARNED FROM PREVIOUS AND ONGOING ERADICATION PROGRAMS?

Two eradication programs that failed (yaws and malaria), one successful program (smallpox), and two ongoing programs that are making excellent progress (dracuncu-

The Eradication of Infectious Diseases
Edited by W.R. Dowdle and D.R. Hopkins © 1998 John Wiley & Sons Ltd.

liasis and poliomyelitis) were reviewed to determine the lessons that can be learned about the societal and political factors that have influenced the outcome of these attempts at disease eradication.

Yaws

The campaign against yaws was one of the early disease control measures initiated by the World Health Organization and conducted from the late 1940s to around 1968. For many African countries south of the Sahara, the period covered the colonial and early independence period when a network of general health services did not exist and the entire government sector could not boast of more than one or two dozens of doctors.

In the African region, the program was introduced to the health authorities who assigned responsibility for its implementation to the mobile teams comprising medical auxiliaries, which were established on the pattern proposed by Jamot in Central Africa in the days of epidemics of trypanosomiasis.

The strategy of control relied on the high sensitivity of the causative organism to injections of the long-acting penicillins. The mobile teams visited the communities in cycles and carried out case-detection and offered treatment. The entire community was treated if the prevalence of the disease exceeded 5% and all juveniles were treated if the prevalence was between 2% and 5%, while only cases and their household contacts were treated if the prevalence was less than 2%. The objective of the yaws campaign was to reduce the prevalence of the disease to such very low levels by repeated visits and treatment until transmission of the disease ceased.

Many countries in the African region of the World Health Organization succeeded in reducing prevalence to levels below 0.5% but discontinued the program prematurely in order to deploy the personnel of the mobile field units to join the static health units established to form the foundation of the newly conceived primary health care (PHC) system to offer continuous care to communities. The result was a resurgence of yaws in almost all of these countries.

There were many reasons for failure of the program, the major reasons being:

1. The epidemiologic assumption that the achievement of low rates of transmission would ultimately interrupt transmission proved incorrect.
2. Global and national priorities shifted away from disease control by mobile teams to service delivery from static facilities.
3. UNICEF and WHO reduced their financial support for yaws eradication.
4. Infected countries lacked the understanding, political commitment, and resources to continue program operation.
5. With decreased emphasis on mobile teams, logistic systems providing penicillin and equipment were disrupted, as were monitoring and evaluation.
6. Parents of children were not informed about the signs of yaws and the need to take infected children for treatment.
7. Many health staff were inadequately trained in the recognition and treatment of yaws cases coming to health facilities.

There were, however, two important legacies of the yaws eradication program:

1. In many countries, the well-trained, motivated mobile teams continued to lead the control of epidemic diseases including smallpox, yellow fever, and meningococcal meningitis.
2. The effectiveness of the "magic" of the penicillin injections in treating pneumonia, sexually transmitted diseases, and infertility created a demand for injections.

Malaria

In the 1950s and 1960s, when the malaria eradication program took place, health infrastructure was in its early stages of development. Policy was established at the global level with implementation through a hierarchical, well-disciplined military-type organization and command structure. Malaria eradication was carried out as a separate, vertical structure that functioned parallel to and in competition with the health system of dispensaries, health posts, and hospitals. This separate program provided geographic mapping, household spraying, case detection, and treatment through protocols that were implemented "by the book" in most countries. Malaria eradication failed for two basic reasons: (1) biologic — as a result of development of vector and parasite drug resistance; and (2) failure of the program to identify and solve problems and utilize findings at the field level to modify strategy. Inadequate attention was given to available scientific evidence suggesting that there was a short time window before insecticide resistance would develop. While the strategy failed, the malaria program provided countries with a number of well-trained, motivated, and disciplined personnel. The malaria eradication program also had the positive effect of demonstrating for the first time that a program could reach virtually every house and every person in the community. Other mass intervention programs which followed based their strategy for extension into the community on the framework developed by malaria workers. Although malaria eradication made major contributions in focusing on the community, the failure of malaria eradication had significant costs in terms of discrediting the concept of disease eradication, questioning the capacity of the health system as a vehicle for technical assistance, and in its failure to strengthen the capacity of the routine health system. The failure of malaria eradication put the concept of eradication under a political shroud for much of the next two decades.

Smallpox

The smallpox eradication program evolved through a collaboration of East (Soviet Union) and West (United States) and involved a unique set of partnerships of noninfected and infected countries. Until 1959, efforts to develop a global consensus for global smallpox eradication were unsuccessful. In that year, Professor Zhdanov of the U.S.S.R. introduced a World Health Assembly resolution calling for global smallpox eradication which passed. Little progress was made, however, until 1966, when again at the impetus of Professor Zhdanov, WHO allocated US$ 2.4 million for eradication. An offer of assistance from the U.S. to the countries in West and Central Africa helped accelerate the program. With strong leadership from WHO, a global coalition of noninfected and infected countries for smallpox eradication was developed. Success resulted from strong technical and management leadership at the global level, the effective mobilization of resources (technical, logistical, financial), and the flexibility to use field data to modify implementation strategies, if appropriate. Another important factor for success was the deliberate use of research for technical innovations, such as the bifurcated needle and heat stable vaccine. The smallpox eradication program learned from the negative experience of malaria the value of training and utilizing health staff *within* the existing health system rather than operating totally independently of it. Its major legacies were the use of field data to evolve operational strategies, culminating in the surveillance and containment strategy, and the development of a cadre of well-trained, motivated field personnel. While the contribution of the smallpox eradication program to infrastructure development was limited, the program provided the framework, foundation, and leadership for the Expanded Program on Immunization (EPI) at local and national levels.

Dracunculiasis

The Guinea worm eradication program is notable for having a strong community-based structure, including village-based volunteers for surveillance purposes, intersectoral collaboration at the district level, and the involvement of nongovernmental organizations in the program, particularly church groups and certain private corporations. Political commitment at the national level has generally been high. A weakness of the program is that the surveillance system, because of its focus on infected areas, has a limited capacity to respond to other national needs for surveillance or to identify unrecognized infected areas (i.e., those missed on original search or new infections). Such a surveillance system shows the need for flexibility, especially in terms of its potential to be adapted for nationwide surveillance for other priority diseases.

Poliomyelitis

The most notable factors favoring the success of the polio eradication program are the constantly improving understanding of the epidemiology of polio, strong contributions to the development of disease surveillance and management capacity within the health services (including creation and ongoing revision of National EPI Plans of Action), development of regional and global laboratory surveillance networks, the achievement of political commitment at the highest levels, the establishment of excellent intersectoral collaboration, and providing the best example of fostering the establishment of interagency coordination committees at the country and regional levels. In addition, the program engendered significant support from the private sector (especially Rotary International) in the form of financial aid, social mobilization, and logistical assistance to the strategic areas of National Immunization Days (NIDs), surveillance, and mop-up immunization activities in high-risk areas.

Major Characteristics of Eradication Programs

Table 14.1 provides a comparison of the major characteristics of these eradication programs. These programs were conducted during differing historical time intervals, encompassing 50 years from the late 1940s to the present, which limits the validity of direct comparisons. Nonetheless, some general trends are illustrated. In general, the more recent eradication programs (dracunculiasis and polio) have benefited from the existence of a more well-developed health infrastructure than was in place during the yaws, malaria, and smallpox eradication programs. Also, there has been an evolution in the process for development of political consensus over time regarding the decision to undertake a disease eradication program. Earlier programs (e.g., malaria, yaws) were characterized by decision-making driven by a select group of experts, sometimes with either official or unofficial endorsement by international organizations such as WHO and the World Health Assembly, and assisted by East–West political solidarity (smallpox). The more recent programs (e.g., dracunculiasis, polio) have incorporated additional efforts to obtain a broader consensus, including the development of North–South consensus and collaboration, development of knowledge and commitment at the highest levels of government, multisectoral collaboration, development of effective systems of communication and surveillance, and establishment of partnerships at the community level.

The structure of the individual programs differs markedly. Factors that positively influence(d) the programs have been divided into the following categories: (1) contribution of the program toward side benefits that improved the health service infrastructure; (2) greater levels of political commitment; (3) the development of intersectoral collaboration; and (4) the extent to which the program engendered interagency support and coordination. Negative program experiences and impacts were also catalogued (last column, Table 14.1). We felt that there is a need to examine further the important roles played by the community, private sector organizations, governmental agencies and the intersectoral collaboration they promote, and the international bilateral and multilateral organizations.

WHAT IS THE ROLE OF COLLABORATING PARTNERS IN DISEASE ERADICATION PROGRAMS?

Effective alliance with all potential collaborators can expand the resource base and enhance the prospects of attaining the objectives of disease eradication initiatives. It was therefore considered necessary to explore ways of promoting the involvement of each collaborating partner and clarify the societal, political, and cultural barriers to eradication.

Table 14.1   Lessons learned from previous eradication programs.

Disease	Period	Existing Health Infrastructure	Program Structure	Contribution to Improve Countries Health Service Infrastructure
Yaws	1940s–1960s	—	Military, strictly vertical	Mobile teams help staffing of fixed health units, introduction of the concept of active surveillance
Malaria	1950s–1960s	+/–	Military, strictly vertical	Geographic mapping and numbering households for regular visiting, leadership
Smallpox	1960s–1970s	+	Surveillance teams, district teams, and community involvement	Surveillance, strategy modification based on field findings, foundation for EPI, leadership training in surveillance, epidemiology, and program management
Dracunculiasis	1980s–1990s	+ +	Community-based, zonal and district support	PHC integrated; village volunteers for surveillance and control measures
Poliomyelitis	1980s–1990s	+ + well-developed EPI within PHC	Existing health service used, NIDs, surveillance developed from day 1	Management and surveillance strengthened, National Plans of Action for EPI, development of line item budget for immunization, increased self-sufficiency in vaccine provision, development and quality control of virological laboratory network

EPI (Expanded Program on Immunization), PHC (Primary Health Care), NIDs (National Immunization Days)

The Community

Several challenges must be addressed to involve the community effectively in a disease eradication program. The first challenge is to generate genuine community partnership rather than simply manipulating the community to do what is required in implementing the disease eradication strategies. By generating such participation, greater sustainable capacity building can occur. A second challenge involves capturing the community's interest and support in balancing the priorities of the global eradication program with those needs that are determined by the community to be important. Since 1985, the experiences in Latin America with social mobilization, in conjunction with the initiative to eradicate polio and strengthen the EPI, provide instructive lessons about building the capacity of the community to make appropriate decisions and to accomplish change for the betterment of the community (PAHO 1996). At the same time,

Table 14.1 *continued*

Disease	Political Commitment	Intersectoral Cooperation	Interagency Cooperation	Negative Program Experience
Yaws	Low political profile of the disease	Only ministry of health involved	Restricted to UNICEF and WHO	Strategies loosely defined, premature dismantling of the program
Malaria	Variable at national level	Minimal	High among limited number of funders	Discredited eradication concept, program failed technically
Smallpox	National leadership in most countries	Minimal	Informal only	Smallpox-focused, short-lived surveillance
Dracunculiasis	Generally strong	Churches and private firms included; also Ministry of Water	Regional interagency coordination group meets annually	Vertical programs, single-purpose community worker
Poliomyelitis	Well developed (especially in Americas) involving top leadership of government and opposition parties; "culture of prevention" established	Well established; private sector strength demonstrated	Interagency Coordination Committees established in all regions, common strategy	Competition between different programs causing community fatigue

UNICEF (United Nations Children's Fund), WHO (World Health Organization)

cooperation was gained to carry out the polio eradication strategies including NIDs and surveillance. An important lesson is the need to develop a more sophisticated understanding by health staff about the most appropriate ways to approach communities and to deal with community development and social organization issues. Another major challenge is how to work in urban communities where community structures may be less well defined.

Private Sector Organizations (non-profit, for-profit)

Private sector involvement has been essential to the dracunculiasis program in terms of DuPont and Precision Fabric Group's contribution of filter material and American Cyanamid's contribution of larvicide. Mobilization of this private sector support has involved advocacy, sharing a vision, documenting the humanitarian impact in terms of human well-being, and working within an understandable time-limited, business-plan framework. We identified the following gaps in knowledge related to the process of getting private sector organizations involved in eradication programs:

1. What factors influence their decision-making process (i.e., what stimulates their interest)?
2. How are decisions made within the organization?
3. How can the priorities and interests of the organization be aligned with the eradication strategies?
4. What are their capacities to provide in kind services?
5. What are their financial capacities?
6. How can the organization's input be properly coordinated at the global, national, and local levels?
7. What are the rewards expected by the organization?
8. What is a reasonable duration of involvement to expect by the organization in the program?
9. What role can the organization play in the political process and advocacy for the program?
10. How much can volunteers be expected to be involved and contribute to the program either on a regular or short-term basis?

Private sector initiatives can be more successful if the government is fully engaged in the disease eradication program.

The example of Rotary International provides a good illustration of the factors that proved instrumental in that organization's decision to become a partner in the polio eradication effort. These factors were as follows (written communication, H. Pigman, Rotary International):

1. Time-limited goal;
2. A humanitarian appeal which resonates well with Rotary's culture of service and volunteerism;
3. The existence of an effective vaccine, which made the goal of polio eradication technically feasible;
4. Agreement by all partners on a global strategy for eradication;
5. The investment factor, i.e., the opportunity for substantial savings in the future as a result of being able to stop vaccinating against polio;
6. A way to support demonstrably cost-effective foreign aid assistance;
7. An emotional factor — the appeal went to people who were "age compatible," namely people of an age who had personal experience with the disease;
8. An effort supportive of broader goals (i.e., the EPI), and an effort which would provide a legacy (better capacity by the health community in fighting infectious diseases);
9. A program that would give the organization good public relations;

10. Participation in intercountry donor aid-coordinating committees, which assured Rotary's knowledge of how its contribution fit into the big picture.

Government/Public Sector Organizations

Important lessons to learn about the public sector are that it responds favorably to: (1) economic saving arguments; (2) a concrete, well-defined goal; (3) the concept of global partnership; (4) the elimination of a disease threat to its own population; (5) a politically attractive program which will show tangible positive impact; and (6) the concept that success in achieving the goal also provides a legacy in the form of improved PHC structure and capacity. To achieve maximum success in a disease eradication program requires not only the involvement of the Minister of Health, but also community and national political leaders (as well as the opposition political party, to avoid any association of the program with a partisan political cause).

Intersectoral Collaboration

One of the most critical lessons affecting the success of a disease eradication program is the importance attached to the development of effective coordinating skills by the Ministry of Health so it can provide leadership in interacting with other Ministries and components of government. Sometimes, such situations can have the unanticipated effect of generating jealousies among other Ministries, however. Effective coordination can attract substantial new resources from outside the health sector without resulting in opportunity costs to other health programs. The increased visibility of the eradication program may increase the likelihood of its achieving a regular budget increase, because of increased recognition regarding its priority relative to other programs outside of the health sector. For example, in the polio eradication program there are a growing number of countries where the increased visibility of the program resulted in the creation by the government of a budget line item that had not previously existed for vaccines for the routine immunization program, or in an increase in the size of the budget in instances where it already existed.

International Organizations (multilateral, bilateral)

These organizations can take a leadership role in the following aspects: (1) to increase the awareness and interest of the global community regarding the global burden of disease of potential candidates for disease eradication initiatives; (2) to disseminate information about the role that disease eradication can play as one of a portfolio of global public health strategies; (3) to play the "gatekeeper" role in formal decision-making and international decision-making; (4) to gather experts and exercise leadership in development of policies and commonly agreed upon strategies; (5) to stimulate the interest and support of national leaders; (6) to coordinate between (among) intercountry and interregional governments in order to facilitate cooperation and joint activities (e.g., fundraising, advocacy, and resource mobilization) at global and country levels.

WHAT IS THE IMPACT AND FUNCTIONAL RELATIONSHIP OF DISEASE ERADICATION AND OTHER TARGETED PROGRAMS ON DEVELOPMENT OF HEALTH INFRASTRUCTURE?

Decision makers at national, regional, and global levels have been challenged to rationalize infrastructural development and community partnerships envisioned by the Conference on Primary Health Care, held at Alma-Ata in 1978, and the focused targets of the 1990 World Summit for Children. There has been a continuing debate as to the impact of disease-specific control programs and disease-specific eradication activities, e.g., polio eradication, on the capacity of the health infrastructure. For the discussion of this topic, we unanimously agreed to look beyond the traditional vertical–horizontal polemic and address two basic questions:

1. What can be learned from our *current* experience about the impact of eradication strategies on health infrastructure (we addressed past experiences in the first section)?
2. How can disease eradication strategies be used to strengthen health system capacity?

The polio and dracunculiasis eradication programs were examined regarding their contributions or lack of contributions to infrastructure development and capacity building.[1] Below is a summary of the major opinions expressed by members of the group.

Positive Impacts of Polio Eradication on Health Infrastructure

1. Development of Interagency Coordinating Committees at regional and country levels.
2. Involvement and commitment of governments (Presidents, Presidents' wives, and opposition politicians).
3. Intersectoral coordination under leadership of government, including:
    *   Development of national plans of action and guidelines,
    *   Improved management capacity and experience, especially in terms of planning, budgeting, monitoring and supervision, logistics,
    *   Mobilization of private for-profit and private nonprofit partnerships,
    *   Development of line item budgets for immunization,
    *   Increased self-sufficiency in vaccine procurement.

---

[1] The only systematic studies we have found that gather data in several countries on the impact of targeted programs on PHC infrastructure were PAHO (1996) and UNICEF (1995b).

4. Development of an effective disease surveillance system and its expansion to surveillance of other diseases of public health importance (e.g., measles, neonatal tetanus, cholera).
5. Development and quality control of regional virological laboratory networks.
6. Enhanced staff capacity (e.g., Western Hemisphere and China); these well-trained health workers have developed additional skills in program management and have contributed to the control of other EPI-targeted diseases.
7. Strengthened commitment to prevention and recognition that vaccination and other preventive services are cost-effective and cost-beneficial.

Negative Impacts of Polio Eradication on Health Infrastructure

1. Focuses on one or a limited number of interventions.
2. Public mobilization for one or a few interventions may represent missed opportunity to address other health priorities.
3. Pressure to achieve results may lead to fabrication of data.
4. Diversion of personnel and resources from other services.
5. Fatigue from repeated NIDs.
6. Transient decreased routine services during NIDs.

Conclusions (Polio)

Regional polio elimination in the Western Hemisphere occurred during a period of social and economic stagnation. Despite these constraints, political advocacy and commitment, regional cooperation, donor support and coordination, and Pan American Health Organization (PAHO) leadership and support facilitated the achievement of polio elimination in the hemisphere. Direct positive cause and effect relationships were most clear for political advocacy, donor coordination, surveillance, and laboratory network development.

Positive Impacts of Dracunculiasis Eradication on Health Infrastructure

1. Focuses on disadvantaged communities.
2. Community centered for surveillance and intervention.
3. Useful in prioritizing installation of safe water supplies.
4. Empowers communities to address their health problems.
5. Addresses economic/social concerns of communities.
6. Increases agricultural production.
7. Increases school attendance.
8. Intersectoral collaboration between Ministers of Health and Ministers of Water.

Negative Impacts of Dracunculiasis on Health Infrastructure

1. Single-purpose community worker.
2. Limited contribution to infrastructure development.
3. High dropout rate of volunteers.
4. Limited use of community resources for other health priorities.

Conclusion (Dracunculiasis)

In general, the principles of dracunculiasis eradication are consistent with and supportive of the principles of PHC.

Recommendations

In looking toward the future of disease eradication programs and their implementation, there was a general consensus that the following principles need to be carefully considered:

1. Eradication programs need to be planned in the context of health services.
2. Eradication programs need to participate in strengthening identified infrastructural and management weaknesses.
3. Resources needed for infrastructure support are inversely proportional to stage of development of the health system. In other words, the least developed systems need the most support (see Table 14.2).

It is recognized that targeted programs (such as eradication of a disease) have been a controversial approach. A continuing controversy is the balancing of global, national, and local priorities to ensure their synergistic and complementary benefits.

The controversy becomes more acute as the implementation of such programs reaches countries with weak infrastructure in the advanced stages of an eradication initiative. It is during this period when the risk of targeting has potential for negative impact on the development of health infrastructure. Therefore, it is important that (a)

Table 14.2 Eradication support to infrastructure development.

Status of Infrastructure	Infrastructure Needs	Risk of Bypassing Capacity Strengthening for Eradication "Quick Fix"	Need for External Resources
Infrastructure well-developed	Focused (e.g., surveillance, planning, management)	Moderate — can be addressed through proper planning as per above	Moderate — can be targeted to specific needs
Infrastructure not well-developed	Enormous (e.g., personnel, equipment, surveillance)	Very high	Very high both in terms of infrastructure and operating costs

global and local priorities be considered and reconciled in the launching of eradication initiatives, and (b) eradication programs be designed so as to support and strengthen existing health infrastructure within the framework of the functional analysis approach presented in Table 14.3.

Integration of eradication activities with PHC has been a stated goal of the functional analysis approach and should be carried out deliberately and systematically; for details of the approach, see Taylor and Waldman (this volume). Particular attention should be paid to balancing top-down and bottom-up functions to prevent difficulties that have sometimes arisen when there was competition between eradication programs

Table 14.3 Analysis of the complementarity among global, national, and local functions (see also UNICEF 1995a).

Global–National–Provincial	District	Social Unit–Community
Program Design, Planning, and Information System		
I. Social mobilization of leaders	Local officials, GO, NGO, religion, business	Community empowerment and self-confidence
II. Equity framework and standards	Performance indicators	Focus on greatest need and most remote areas
III. Surveillance and monitoring framework	Response capability	Reporting
IV. Periodic evaluation	Continuing monitoring and evaluation	Community-based Self-evaluation with Essential Data (SEED)
V. Priority definition global	Regional priority	Local priority
VI. Financing for global priority	Distribution with equity	Self-financing for local priorities without dependency
Implementation		
I. Framework for "going to scale" with national extension	Training and experimentation centers for regional extension	Testing and adapting local level "minimum packages of care"
II. Training of trainers	Training of local workers	Education for community capacity building
III. Supervision framework and technical assistance	Supportive supervision	Community-based supervision
IV. Selection of scientific knowledge that is appropriate for local conditions	Regional expertise to adapt scientific interventions to local reality	Capacity building to integrate simplified scientific knowledge with local understanding of what works
V. Logistics and transportation	Maintenance	Local maintenance
VI. Framework for quality control and standards	Performance indicators and assessment	Flexible adaptation capacity

and other services. If eradication programs are appropriately integrated, the long-term sustainability of improvements in health infrastructure should be enhanced and will facilitate eradication goals. Table 14.3 lists six functions in planning and program design, and six in implementation. The matrix shows how responsibility for particular components of each function can be allocated differently to central, district, and community levels. The community component is especially important for activities requiring social mobilization. For example, it is essential to generate community cooperation to achieve high levels of coverage in NIDs. The functional analysis approach provides a framework for such collaboration.

WHAT ARE THE TRENDS AFFECTING HEALTH DEVELOPMENT THAT WILL INFLUENCE ERADICATION PROGRAMS IN THE FUTURE?

Our group discussed in broad terms some of the global trends that can have an impact, either positively or negatively, on future disease eradication efforts. The major points are summarized below.

Globalization

Noted were trends toward global centralization in areas such as information to the public (e.g., satellite communication); increasing financial power vested in ever larger commercial conglomerates; regional political and economic alliances (e.g., European Union); and the consequent vesting of power in fewer and fewer hands. Such trends can be positive factors if intelligently exploited by the health community. For example, the sense of "corporate citizenship" can be applied, particularly if the appeal can demonstrate economic benefits (e.g., reduction in work days lost through illness and disability), as well as general improvement in community health. The news media can help raise awareness of health concerns and priorities in a way that can influence political action.

Demographics

Particularly in poorer countries, population growth offers a continuing challenge to the PHC system to keep pace with the needs. Such countries need continuing donor support in their efforts to establish sustainable health systems. When such countries embark on a coordinated global eradication program, they will need assurances of donor support to supplement what may be meager national resources. Countries with well-established systems can carry most or all of the burden of special eradication costs; countries with weak systems must rely on a high percentage of outside resources. It is recognized that increasing life expectancies achieved through preventive health care have the long-term effect of reducing birth rates, especially if health and family planning services are integrated.

Equity

The process of globalization, particularly in relation to trade and information, has brought into play new factors in the international relationships that have an important impact on health. For example, the increased communication and contact among nations and communities has increased the possibility of transmission of infectious diseases across borders. Another factor is that with the increased control of resources by global enterprises, the gap between rich and poor has widened, bringing about substantial inequalities in health among different population groups. Collectively, these two factors have had a negative impact on the health of populations in developing and developed countries alike. One health strategy that can help bring about health equity is the eradication of a disease, which has the effect of reaching the entire population to improve equity and social justice.

Decentralization

Many governments are decentralizing health management responsibility to the district and local levels. Decentralization of health services is giving the local community much greater control of how health funds are deployed. Thus, good communication will be essential in future eradication programs in order to secure participation and commitment at provincial, county, township and village levels. The "packaging" of a global objective with a health objective of regional or local concern may be useful in achieving success, as well as greater cost-effectiveness. While the process of decentralization has increased the ownership and responsibilities of local communities and governments, with the potential for mobilization of additional resources, it also has the potential to affect adversely those communities with the fewest resources. Decentralization should not stop at the district level but be extended effectively and equitably to the community. Moreover, there is also the potential to disrupt the capacity of national level authorities to perform certain functions (e.g., disease surveillance). Provided this devolution is accompanied by allocation of adequate resources, local authorities are well-positioned to mobilize local political support and resources to provide a balanced approach to national and local priorities.

Privatization

The democratization of governments that has occurred in recent years in several countries throughout the world has favored a process of health care reform in which a major feature is the privatization of the health services. While these processes have brought new partners into the financing of health services, there is a tendency in these new schemes to favor the financing of curative health care, with preventive medicine not having a high profile in many countries. Another potential negative impact of privatization on health is that the research and development of new vaccines and drugs is almost entirely in the private sector, which does not necessarily ensure that many diseases which are most prevalent in developing countries will be targeted for vaccine or drug development.

Economics

As the global economy grows, so does the gap between rich and poor. Eradication programs offer an outstanding example of how rich and poor nations can team up to achieve direct benefits to both. For example, the polio eradication program brings lasting benefits and reaches the most disadvantaged, the poorest of the poor, in financially distressed societies. At the same time, the program will produce significant savings to all collaborating nations. The same was true for the smallpox eradication program.

Peace

It can be expected that the world will be plagued with continuing civil and regional conflicts, the result of a reemergence of long-suppressed regional and ethnic animosities which previously had been kept in check during the "Cold War" era. "Days of Tranquility," in which combatants declare a cease-fire for such events as polio NIDs or dracunculiasis eradication activities, should continue to be used and may even have value in contributing toward more lasting peace and understanding of common interests (Hull 1997; CDC 1995).

Resources for Development

Regrettably, overseas development aid provided by wealthy donor nations is decreasing in magnitude, reaching an average of 0.3% of GNP in 1994, the lowest level in 20 years (Report of the Organization for Economic Cooperation and Development 1996). This trend must be reversed by concerted efforts, stressing the cost-effectiveness of preventive health care and interventions such as vaccines.

Progress in Medical Science and Technology

The development of new and improved vaccines, drug therapies, vector control, and other preventive approaches will contribute substantially to the prospects for considering future eradication programs.

MOVING FROM DISEASE CONTROL TO DISEASE ERADICATION: WHAT ARE THE ESSENTIAL SOCIETAL AND POLITICAL CRITERIA?

An eradication program requires major human and financial resources as well as political will to be successful. Hence, the success of a disease eradication initiative, like any public health program, is largely dependent on the level of societal and political commitment to it from beginning to end. While disease eradication is now established as a public health strategy, the potentially enormous costs of failure dictate that any proposal for eradication be given intense scrutiny. Thus, understanding the process of developing and maintaining political and societal consensus is critical to the success of the eradication program. We have reviewed many of the factors involved in this process and offer the following sequential framework for considering the political and societal factors which influence success or failure.

Justifying the Need for an Eradication Program

The disease under consideration for eradication must be of recognized public health importance, engender broad international appeal for undertaking its eradication, and be perceived as a significant problem by the population, ideally at all levels of society from the global level to the community. The disease must be documented to be a major cause of morbidity, mortality, and/or disability, and a significant economic burden to society. Unless the burden of disease and economic impact are sufficient to be clearly appreciated and to generate political will and popular support, there is the danger that national financial support for the program will not be forthcoming or continuing.

There should be a specific reason for eradication, rather than control, of the disease. The demand for sustained, high-quality performance and perseverance in an eradication program runs the danger of failure with consequent significant loss of credibility, financial loss, and erosion of morale and self-confidence of health workers. Therefore, a specific reason for pursuing eradication instead of control is needed to justify the calculated risk involved (e.g., the ability to stop vaccination against the disease). When progress in the control of the disease has reached a plateau, and the application of reasonable additional resources, for a limited period, offers assurance of achieving the goal of eradication and thus capturing from future savings the cost of the special intervention, a critical threshold is exceeded favoring the eradication of the disease.

Assessing the Feasibility of Eradication

A technically feasible intervention and eradication strategy has to be identified, field tested in a defined geographic area, and found effective. Momentum needs to be generated from the accumulation of success in individual countries or within a region, building in such a way as to advance political will. Economic analysis at this stage shows eradication to be a good investment in development.

Gaining Consensus

Consensus review by technical experts (health and social scientists, planners) must justify the priority for eradication of the disease. Education of decision makers as to the need, possibilities and costs must take place. In addition, the scientific community must be educated and enlisted. Global, national, and local priorities need to be considered and reconciled in anticipation of the launching of the eradication initiative.

Making the Decision

Political commitment must be obtained at the highest levels, following informed discussion at regional and global levels. A clear commitment of resources from international sources is essential at the start.

The final decision-making process must include passage of a resolution on disease eradication by the World Health Assembly. The background information needed for such a resolution should include: (a) the main implications for the countries themselves (e.g., enhanced surveillance, establishment or improvement of lab network, need for NIDs, etc.), including time frame for individual activities and anticipated resource requirements, and (b) to the extent possible, an estimated global and regional budget.

Developing Support

An advocacy plan must be prepared and ready for full implementation at global, regional, and national levels. An effective alliance with all potential collaborators and partners should be in operation. Recruitment of partners and coordination of resources through interagency coordination committee activities at the national, regional, and global levels is essential. It is also necessary to be able to persuade all affected countries to commit to implementing the eradication intervention(s) and maintaining them within a defined period of time. The eradication program should address the issue of inequity and be supportive of broader goals that positively impact on the health infrastructure and provide an additional legacy besides the eradication of the disease.

Implementation within the Framework of the Health System

1. The eradication program needs to be planned in the context of health services.
2. The eradication program needs to participate in strengthening identified infrastructural and management weaknesses.
3. Resources needed for infrastructure support are inversely proportional to stage of development of the health system. In other words, the least developed systems will need the most support.
4. Eradication programs should be designed so as to support and strengthen existing health infrastructure, using a functional approach that balances global, national, and local priorities.

Sequencing Eradication Efforts

The political and societal momentum gained by a successful eradication initiative is an important element for phasing in another eradication effort. For example, long before the goal of polio eradication was achieved in the Western Hemisphere, political authorities of countries which had successfully reached the goal were pressing to move into regional elimination of measles to capitalize on the gains made by the previous polio eradication program. The sequencing approach not only made it possible to secure continuing political commitment and financing for immunization programs, it also facilitated the sustainment of the disease surveillance system at a level adequate to comply with the stringent requirements of an eradication program long after the last detected case occurred.

REFERENCES

CDC (Centers for Disease Control and Prevention). 1995. Implementation of health initiatives during a cease-fire: Sudan, 1995. *Morbid. Mortal. Wkly. Rep.* **44(23)**:433–436.

Hull, H.F. 1997. Pax polio. *Science* **275**:40–41.

PAHO (Pan American Health Organization). 1996. The Impact of the Expanded Program on Immunization and the Polio Eradication Initiative on Health Systems in the Americas. Final Report of the Taylor Commission. Washington, D.C.: PAHO.

Report of the Organization for Economic Cooperation and Development. 1996. Paris: OECD Communications Divisions.

UNICEF (United Nations Children's Fund). 1995a. Community-based Sustainable Human Development — Going to Scale with Self-Reliant Social Development. UNICEF Environment Section. New York: UNICEF.

UNICEF. 1995b. Sustainability of Achievements, Lessons Learned from Universal Child Immunization. Steering Committee chaired by Marc LaForce. New York: UNICEF.

15

Are There Better Global Mechanisms for Formulating, Implementing, and Evaluating Eradication Programs?

I. ARITA

Agency for Cooperation in International Health (ACIH), 4–11–1 Higashi-machi,
Kumamoto City, 862 Japan

ABSTRACT

The success of global smallpox eradication and the subsequent successful initiation of polio eradication in the Americas have signaled a departure from the past failure of eradication efforts against yellow fever, yaws, and malaria.

It is now believed that eradication of a few vaccine-preventable diseases as well as some tropical diseases should take place as a special and newly emerging global effort in the 21st century. New technological developments could accelerate this process.

Past experiences have shown that several eradication or elimination efforts were not initiated with a full understanding of the target diseases. Also, the globally coordinated efforts were insufficient in terms of social and political commitment. These were some of the reasons for the failure of past programs. In view of the fact that to initiate, implement, and assess future eradication or elimination efforts requires substantial research and coordination of efforts on a global scale, there should be a newly established mechanism to promote such development. It is proposed that such a mechanism would best function if a special program were developed within the World Health Organization (WHO) or elsewhere in the United Nations' (UN) system.

Because of the complexities of eradication, this chapter proposes the creation of such a special mechanism. Establishment of a vaccine fund, laboratory network, and research are also discussed as they are important elements in the eradication process.

INTRODUCTION

The lessons learned from the successful eradication of smallpox are twofold. First, several biological criteria favored its success, namely lack of an animal reservoir, lack

The Eradication of Infectious Diseases
Edited by W.R. Dowdle and D.R. Hopkins © 1998 John Wiley & Sons Ltd.

of persistent infection, availability of an effective tool, and world interest (Arita 1979). The second lesson is broader, namely humankind was able to unify its efforts for eradication of a disease despite vast differences among participating nations in terms of politics, religion, race, and culture. The presently successful program for polio eradication in the Western Hemisphere, I believe, corroborates these lessons.

In this chapter, I review a few practical problems, taking into account the lessons mentioned above so that future eradication programs may be better planned, implemented, and certified.

PERMANENT EFFECTS OF ERADICATION

The clear difference between eradication and control of infectious diseases is that an eradication program, when it succeeds, can result in the disestablishment of all control measures. This advantage is of paramount importance not only from the viewpoint of cost effectiveness but also because it completely alters the traditional concept of humans fighting against diseases. In other words, eradication includes not only interruption of disease transmission in the human population but also the disestablishment of all the public health measures that were maintained until eradication was achieved. Additionally, it would be ideal to destroy laboratory stocks of the causative agents. This latter step, however, may become increasingly difficult as in the future, science may become able to create the causative agents or there will be a number of institutions having such special agents, all of which would not be known, making complete destruction difficult.

In the case of smallpox eradication, for example, destruction of smallpox virus stocks in WHO Collaborating Centers in Atlanta and Novosibirsk is scheduled for 1999. This would complete the annihilation of that pathogen from the surface of the earth. One may argue that the destruction of such virus stocks might cause a disadvantage, namely losing important biological research material in the future. In my view, however, there is presently a more real danger of the virus escaping through human error or terrorism into the totally unimmunized world population (we stopped vaccination in 1980), and such danger exceeds the research benefit mentioned above.

Thus, eradication is definitely a superior method of fighting against disease, compared to the usual control methods. Richard Doll mentioned that the 21st century would be the era of preventive medicine (Doll 1982). This consideration may be further endorsed by the prospect that in the 21st century, target diseases for eradication may be increased because of better vaccines, treatments (reducing source of infection), and other technological developments, making eradication a newly emerging strategy to deal with infectious diseases (Arita 1997).

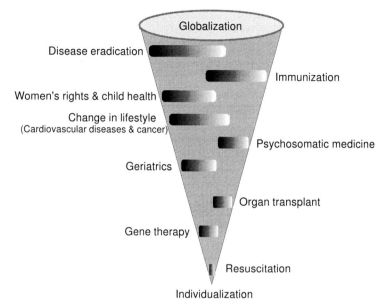

Figure 15.1 Global eradication is a logical consequence of the evolution of medical technology in the mainstream of globalization of the 21st centruy. Note this is contrasted by the revival in the trend of individualization on the other extreme end.

BEGINNING OF ERADICATION EFFORTS

The history of eradicating human diseases can be traced back to the various programs which began in the first half of this century. The major eradication efforts included yellow fever, yaws, malaria, and smallpox. Only smallpox eradication succeeded. All were motivated by scientific idealism. None of them, however, appears to have started with a fully comprehensive assessment of feasibility of eradication or understanding of the epidemiology of the target disease. My personal experiences in smallpox eradication indicate that although the program started with a WHO Assembly's resolution in 1958, the program became effective only in 1967, when intensified efforts were introduced by a renewed WHO Assembly resolution (1966) coupled with a large investment of WHO's regular budget and the creation of a new WHO unit for smallpox eradication. Till then, it was naively believed that mass vaccination programs being conducted by the national health administrations of individual endemic countries could eliminate the disease. Further it was thought that the program could be implemented by endemic countries with their own resources, although the U.S.S.R. offered vaccine to the global program.

This Intensified Global Smallpox Eradication Program made three basic improve-ments: assurance of vaccine quality, introduction of epidemiological surveillance, and containment vaccination in the immediate areas or community where effective sur-veillance discovered transmission of the disease. I would note that at that time there was considerable resistance by member states to approve the 1966 WHO Assembly Resolution. For example, in the Assembly, the proposed budget to intensify the smallpox eradication program was accepted by a margin of two votes; the narrowest margin in the history of WHO. Such resistance was influenced by the failing malaria eradication program at that time.

Thus, even the successful smallpox eradication program experienced a great deal of difficulty at the onset of the intensified program. An eradication program should not be undertaken without comprehensive analysis of its feasibility in terms of biological, social, and political conditions.

Currently, the global polio eradication program is under way. The program, however, was conducted for five years in the Western Hemisphere, under the leadership of the Pan American Health Organization (PAHO), before it expanded, eight years after the certification of smallpox in 1980. Thus the program did not start with a global agreement. Parenthetically, the reason for such late commencement of polio eradication was influenced by the fear of many policymakers, namely that another specific disease-targeted program might interfere with the development of basic health services. The polio eradication program in the Western Hemisphere was successful (last case in Peru in 1991 and certification in 1994) but will have to wait for the certification in the Eastern Hemisphere, which is expected at the earliest in 2003 or 2004. Until then, countries in the Western Hemisphere will have to continue surveillance as well as immunizations. This results from different policy decisions in different WHO regions, leading to less cost effectiveness in the overall eradication efforts. Measles eradication has also now started in the Americas, but not yet in other WHO regions. Again, a similar course of events might occur.

These historical reviews on the beginning of eradication programs make us think; we need to study the critical factors for initiation of eradication efforts in the future.

FACTORS TO CONSIDER IN INITIATING ERADICATION EFFORTS

First, *the real meaning of eradication is not often understood by many policymakers, scientists, and the public.* When I was in the program of smallpox eradication, public health officers often stated: "Yes, smallpox can be eradicated, but after eradication, where is smallpox?" At that time, a high official of WHO mentioned at a WHO meeting that the eradication of smallpox could be completed, but that it was still alright if the disease just remained in some remote areas in the world. It is most important that the meaning of eradication should be understood, since the program requires full global support politically and socially. It should also be noted that the permanent effect of eradication has been shown by the fact that smallpox does not return even if all health infrastructures have been destroyed, as for example, in Liberia, Somalia, Rwanda, Brundi, and Bosnia.

Second, *feasibility studies should be comprehensively carried out.* Despite the bright scope of eradication, as mentioned above, its initiation should be managed with utmost care so that we will not repeat the failure of eradication in the past. Potential target diseases, as mentioned above, include, in my opinion, polio, measles, rubella, hepatitis B, diphtheria, dracuncliasis, and lymphatic filariasis. The feasibility of eradicating (or eliminating) these diseases will have to be evaluated in terms of (a) biological characteristics of target diseases, (b) social and political commitment, (c) global mobilization of resources, and (d) of technical judgment so that after eradication all nations can stop the control measures. It would be an enormous job to sort out the feasibility and coordinate global agreement for launching the efforts.

Third, *for future programs, concern has been expressed by a few health planners that eradication efforts may hamper the development of basic health services.* This should be fully discussed and a sensible solution has to be sought. The resistance encountered by the member states when the renewed Intensified Smallpox Eradication Program began in 1967 was based on this fear. I am not an expert on primary health care development but would like to add my experience in smallpox eradication: this eradication program, contrary to the concern, actually helped to *strengthen* basic health services. The national smallpox eradication program in Somalia, late in 1970, provides one such example. The program started in the areas where no census data and no health infrastructure existed. The successful campaign resulted in the availability of demographic data and development of rudimentary health service system in rural areas. (Unfortunately, these were destroyed by recent civil war.)

This is a positive example; however, a negative example occurs when a few eradicable diseases are being handled simultaneously by health services. For example, when polio eradication started in the WHO region of the Western Pacific, a few national programs had to handle polio eradication, measles immunization, and neonatal tetanus elimination program at the same time. This caused problems of prioritization and, in fact, led to confusion.

MEETING REQUIREMENTS TO INITIATE GLOBAL ERADICATION OR ELIMINATION OF DISEASES IN THE 21st CENTURY

As mentioned in the foregoing sections, the situation is complex, and if the world health community really wishes to initiate and successfully implement these global programs, we need to handle the global programs systematically and with enhanced analytical capability.

In my opinion, a practical way to achieve better results would be to set up a new global program unit for disease eradication within WHO or the UN to analyze, promote, and execute global eradication of candidate diseases. I raise the choice of two organizations — the WHO or UN — to avoid rigidity in the proposal, as the scope of global activities in the 21st century might have rather large implications in terms of political and social commitment. The UN AIDS program is an example. Needless to say, if WHO member states willingly take up these tremendous programs, WHO would be the organization of first choice as its constitution includes the eradication of diseases as a mandate.

It may be useful for private foundations — which in principle are politically independent and with minimal bureaucracy have access to the best advisors (as being done by Dahlem Konferenzen in Berlin) — to organize special reviews on various criteria. However, such reviews would have a limited impact because they cannot promote the global political will to act. For such a global program, all the nations will need to participate without exception. Such being the case, it is logical to propose the establishment of a special program unit, either within WHO or in UN, to handle the promotion of global eradication programs.

THE FUNCTIONS OF A WHO OR UN UNIT FOR ERADICATION OF SPECIAL DISEASES

These would be as follows:

- to analyze the feasibility of eradication regarding candidate diseases (biological, social/political, financial, and certification), undertaking necessary research,
- to prepare for global implementation, which will be done if the disease shows good feasibility,
- to assist the implementation, which will be done mainly by national programs,
- to coordinate such activities in collaboration with nongovernmental organizations (NGOs) and bilateral agencies,
- to evaluate progress,
- to secure appropriate resources, and
- to certify whether eradication is achieved.

Major organizational divisions might include: (1) general management, (2) strategic planning, (3) technology development and implementation, including laboratory aspects of the program, (4) evaluation, (5) supply and equipment, (6) information, (7) research, and (8) fund raising.

If the system is part of WHO, the current WHO regional structure would be used. If it consists of another UN agency, such an organization should be located at a center of world air traffic. There would be a head office in Geneva and four regional offices, for example one each in Washington, D.C., New Delhi, Beijing, and Cairo. These locations are tentative, but give some idea of how this might be approached.

SPECIAL REMARKS ON PLANNING AND EXECUTING VACCINE PROCUREMENT

Target diseases for future eradication efforts will be vaccine-preventable diseases such as measles, rubella, hepatitis B, and diphtheria.

From the experiences gained during the global smallpox and polio eradication programs, we see that in the first three to four years, there were severe shortages of or difficulties in obtaining a supply of vaccine (production capacity, quality, and timely supply). In fact, WHO, UNICEF, the various national programs, and NGOs spent enormous time and effort just simply to secure an adequate vaccine supply. Quality was also a problem. In the case of smallpox eradication, only 30% of manufacturers met WHO's standard over the first few years (Arita 1972). I propose that there should be special "vaccine funds" with which a limited number of manufacturers can enjoy economical production on long-term basis. This could serve to make the price of vaccine affordable. Quality control would be also easier. It should be noted that polio, as well as measles, vaccine will not be needed once eradication is achieved; thus these vaccines have a short life. This implication influences the investment method in the production of certain vaccines, i.e., resources are allocated to the production of vaccines with long life, as opposed to short life.

International Reference Laboratories

It may be necessary to set up a limited number of diagnostic laboratories. As smallpox or polio eradication has shown, surveillance is the key to success, and surveillance must depend upon a reliable laboratory diagnosis network with effective management. Very often, such laboratory development will be delayed. There should be international collaborating laboratories which would assist in establishing the national laboratories. The number of such laboratories (either collaborating or national) should be limited so that each lab can develop its reliability with a sufficient number of test specimens, and thus avoiding dispersed resource allocation. During the last phase of the smallpox eradication program, all the specimens collected by national programs worldwide were sent to the WHO headquarters in Geneva, which dispatched them to only two WHO collaborating centers for smallpox eradication: in Atlanta and Moscow. These are rather extreme measures but they assured rapidity and reliability of laboratory tests. At that time, each laboratory tested about 5000 specimens per year (WHO 1980).

The Length of Time for Eradication and Leadership

The duration of an eradication program should not be too long, perhaps in the range of 10–15 years. The programs will have to be a "crash" type, supported by unified efforts of individual nations, NGO, and donors. If the period is too long, cost effectiveness will be reduced. Also, it is difficult to sustain a high level of enthusiasm throughout the period.

It is often said that the disease will disappear sooner or later in the course of economic development resulting in better hygiene and medical services. The concept of eradication, however, emphasizes the importance of the time factor. Because eradication has a time limit, it becomes useful in terms of the cost benefit. For example, poliomyelitis incidence might become zero toward the end of 21st century as almost all nations might have achieved by then good immunization programs. The reason for placing importance on global polio eradication now is its time limit, namely the eradication by the year 2000. As the ending time is prolonged, usefulness of eradication efforts diminish.

Such a time-limited program requires strong leadership. That leadership needs a clearly defined target, and eradication can provide this. The success of smallpox eradication was due to WHO's leadership and national program leaders. WHO's Intensified Program for Smallpox Eradication sometimes did not follow its own conventional rules. For example, all communication was supposed to go through regional offices, but the program sometimes established direct contact with national programs for urgent action required because of intense epidemics.

Research

Despite meticulous analysis and planning, some new technical discovery can occur during a eradication program. In yellow fever eradication, e.g., it is well known that the discovery of an animal reservoir of yellow fever virus destroyed hope of eradication. In smallpox eradication, discovery of human monkeypox in West and Central Africa in 1970s caused the suspicion that smallpox could also have an animal reservoir, but ten years of surveillance and virological research concluded that human monkeypox should not frustrate the eradication of smallpox (Arita et al. 1985).

Thus, it is vitally important for research activities (biological, epidemiological, and operational) to be a part of eradication efforts. Research funds must be secured, and researchers encouraged.

Special Remarks on Resources

It is notable that one of the methods for fund raising is to attract the interest of child health-related industries (such as toys, games, baby food/children's food, etc.). In Japan, the Agency for Cooperation in International Health, where I am affiliated, contacted about 50 such industries in Japan; ten showed interest since they felt they must do something good for children. We are now trying to organize such interested industries into one special committee so that they may participate in important Japanese and global programs. Global eradication of a few childhood infectious diseases may be one of the ideal target programs which may attract their interest. Since newborn and young children are immediately exposed to such infectious diseases, eradication of such diseases would be very good; after all, its effect is forever.

CAN ERADICATION EFFORTS BE COUPLED WITH ELIMINATION PROGRAMS FOR TROPICAL DISEASES?

Considering the major task for eradicating more than five diseases (vaccine preventable) in the 21st century, it would seem logical to set up the special mechanism

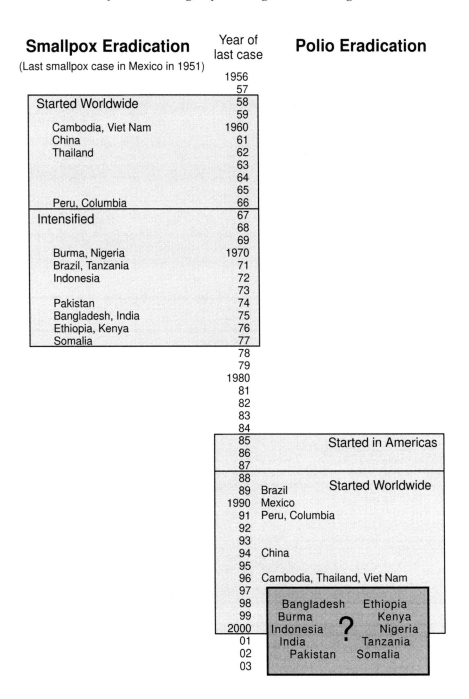

Figure 15.2 Comparison of two global programs a with 10- to 15-year time frame for eradication.

mentioned in previous sections. The preparation for this should start in the near future. The question arises as to whether such a system can include the current WHO's elimination initiative of dracunculiasis (already initiated), onchocerciasis, lymphatic filariasis, and Chagas disease. My answer is "yes." Although control measures against these tropical diseases are different from vaccine-preventable diseases, there are some common features requiring (1) operation on a global or continental basis, (2) intensive disease specific operation with surveillance, and (3) aims to reduce the incidence to zero (eradication) or to very minimum level (elimination). Thus, joint work would be more beneficial. After all, at the peripheral level, a few target diseases will have to be handled by the same health infrastructure.

Expansion of eradication programs for vaccine-preventable diseases to include elimination of tropical diseases would further stimulate the concept that eradication is not just a handful of enthusiastic people but a program in which much broader public and private circles should participate. I believe that such a program could become a new category of public health activity in the 21st century.

REFERENCES

Arita, I. 1972. The control of vaccine quality in the smallpox eradication programme. In: International Symposium on Smallpox Vaccine, Bilthovern, The Netherlands, Oct. 11–13, 1972. Symposia Series in Immuno-biological Standardization, vol. 19, pp. 78–87. Basel: Karger.

Arita, I. 1979. Virological evidence for the success of the smallpox eradication programme. *Nature* **279(5711)**:293–298.

Arita, I. 1997. The prospect for use of preventive medicine in developing countries. *Environ. Sci.* **4(S001–S006)**:1–6. Tokyo: MYU.

Arita, I., Z. Jezek, et al. 1985. Human monkeypox: A newly emerged orthopox virus zoonosis in the tropical rain forest of Africa. *Am. J. Trop. Med. Hyg.* **34**:781–789.

Doll, R. 1982. Prospects for Prevention, the Harveian Oration. London: Royal College of Physicians.

WHO (World Health Organization). 1980. Final Report of the Global Commission for the Certification of Smallpox Eradication. Geneva: WHO.

16

Thoughts on Organization for Disease Eradication

W. FOEGE

Dept. of International Health, The Rollins School of Public Health of Emory University,
1518 Clifton Rd., NE, 7th Floor, Atlanta, GA 30322, U.S.A.

INTRODUCTION

What is needed to improve our global approach and organization for eradication? What do we need to know in order to make a decision to pursue eradication? If eradication appeared to be sensible and justifiable, how would the scientific community be constructively mobilized to make that case? What social and political steps would be needed? How would resources be secured and how could the world organize, both to examine such questions and to accomplish the goal?

MAKING THE CASE

Health programs, in general, start with the obligation to do no harm. While health programs would like to have only benefits and no risks or harmful effects, rarely is that hope achievable. In practice, therefore, health programs attempt to minimize harm, try exceedingly hard to have the benefits far outweigh the risks, and put great resources into reducing the risk. At times, society accepts, consciously, the risk to a few (as in polio vaccine-associated paralysis) as a price worth paying for the benefits to many.

Advocates of eradication programs should insist on a high burden of proof that includes:

- Making the case for the reductions in suffering and premature death expected to result from eradication. Increasingly, measures such as *disability adjusted life years* (DALY) or *quality life years* (QALY) can be used to assess the burden of disease resulting from an organism or other condition.
- Demonstrating an acceptable return on investment as compared to other health activities (cost per DALY, etc.). It is also important to agree on the time period since eradication benefits continue forever.

The Eradication of Infectious Diseases
Edited by W.R. Dowdle and D.R. Hopkins © 1998 John Wiley & Sons Ltd.

- Demonstrating the benefits in terms of development.
- Demonstrating the benefits to the strengthening of the health infrastructure. How will eradication have health benefits beyond the disease targeted? That is, what are the expectations that the eradication effort will act as a tugboat for other health activities rather than a sandbar to block other actions?
- An understanding of the risks or harm associated with the program and a demonstration that these are small and far exceeded by the benefits.

SCIENTIFIC CAPACITY AND SOCIAL WILL

Eradication programs are only possible if the science exists to interrupt disease transmission permanently. It is important to determine whether the science exists or whether there are clear steps that can be taken to make the science adequate to the task. Because scientific abilities improve so rapidly, it is important to have frequent reviews of what might be possible in terms of disease eradication based on recent innovations, as well as a frequent review of the latest thinking on barriers to eradication and the research indicated to surmount those barriers. The review accomplished by the Task Force for Disease Eradication has provided a great first step (CDC 1993). This needs to be reexamined periodically.

Elaborate new structures are probably not needed to accomplish such reviews. Past and current activities (including this workshop) demonstrate the interest that exists. Scientists at, e.g., the World Health Organization (WHO), National Institutes of Health (NIH), and Centers for Disease Control and Prevention (CDC) examine their own fields on a continuing basis because of the interest they have in judging how far the science can be pushed. What is needed is a point of responsibility to maintain an informal network, to provide a vision of disease eradication that crosses all fields of interest, and to promote activities that would not be undertaken by a single disease field. Such an informal network could make sure reviews are done on a frequent basis, could determine where additional research is needed and promote such research, and could organize workshops or special meetings to pursue promising ideas in more detail.

In short, the science capacity for analysis of eradication possibilities exists and needs only to be coordinated. The much more difficult issue involves how to organize efforts to achieve eradication.

ORGANIZATION FOR ERADICATION

The world is in its infancy in developing global organization mechanisms. Fifty years of experience is insufficient to know what works in the long run, or to have experience with alternative approaches. Therefore the subject should be approached with humility and flexibility. Several observations seem pertinent.

1. The involvement of WHO is necessary but insufficient for an eradication campaign. A cursory glance at past efforts indicates that with smallpox eradication, resistance to accept this challenge at WHO was overcome only with considerable outside help. The collaboration of the U.S.S.R. and the U.S.A. was an essential part of the effort. The contributions in people and resources from CDC were also important ingredients.

2. With polio eradication, WHO resisted the opportunity to be involved until the World Health Assembly, in May, 1988, passed a resolution on eradication. That resolution, in turn, was the result of much work and deliberate education of health ministries, accomplished outside of the organization to encourage them to accept the responsibility. To the credit of WHO, once the resolution passed, they took the lead. The point of importance here is that leadership for developing a global polio eradication effort (which began in the Pan American Health Organization) then went outside of WHO before it reached such compelling strength that it could be easily accepted by the Organization. The lesson may be that WHO should be seen as a scientific organization that becomes an eradication advocate only when outside forces are sufficiently strong to make the case. That may not be a bad model to follow in the future.

3. Eradication of dracunculiasis (Guinea worm disease) was actively resisted by WHO, and it is fair to say that they warmed to the campaign only when it appeared to be bound for success. The bottom line is that WHO's involvement is important and WHO leadership is desired; however, that is not enough. Furthermore, the experience to date suggests that eradication efforts would not be at their current level if WHO had to *initiate* the effort. Again, the lesson from Guinea worm eradication may be that the best approach may well be to promote efforts outside the WHO until efforts reach a critical mass both scientifically and socially that is comfortable for their embrace. It may be a mistake to accept the delays inherent in expecting WHO to provide the early leadership.

4. Health leadership now and in the future will depend on those who can develop networks and coalitions. It is no longer possible for a person to organize a successful global health effort just because of their title. It requires so many partnerships of private, public, nongovernmental organizations (NGOs), donor, service and volunteer groups that no single organization or structure can be expected to carry out all eradication efforts.

5. Experience to date makes the above point more than theoretical. Smallpox eradication was directed by WHO but included significant help from CDC, USAID, other bilaterals, and the private sector (including the Wyeth patent). Polio has now developed a great coalition. Indeed, the activities and the organization provide a model of ways to combine interests. However, the catalytic role was played by a service organization, Rotary International. Guinea worm eradication has been totally dependent on an NGO, the Carter Center. Onchocerciasis, if added to the eradication list, will have been energized by a corporation, the Merck Company, Inc. A lesson from this is to avoid a

single organization concept and be prepared to do the necessary work to create a tailor-made structure for each eradication effort. This requires utilizing the capabilities now available in the global, national, and local health organizations, asking what is needed to fill the interstices, and calculating how to use the eradication organization to strengthen the infrastructure for other health activities.

Given the above observations, one could conclude that the expectation of WHO as a site for disease eradication ferment is misplaced. Furthermore, the development of a separate UN global organization for disease eradication would be expensive, could be divisive and competitive, and would probably reduce the opportunity for innovation with new disease problems. In fact, it might well eventually reduce the ability to contemplate eradication efforts by stifling innovation.

Instead, a less formal method is desirable, to provide a mechanism for examining possible disease eradication targets, based on a network of interested scientists. The network would review current scientific possibilities, determine research opportunities for surmounting barriers to eradication, and when feasible, make the scientific and economic case for pursuing an eradication program. Actual eradication plans would then be developed to determine how best to organize and coordinate the many public, private, and other groups who could potentially be involved. It is likely that as in the past, a different organization would evolve for each effort, the common theme being the utilization and strengthening of the current health infrastructure in each country.

A LARGER CONTEXT

Finally, the vision for disease eradication should go beyond the elimination of a disease. The spread of democracy in many countries in recent years has made clear that experience is important in developing democratic processes as well as confidence in the process. For example, the U.S. experimented for over a century before giving women the right to vote! That seems almost unreal in hindsight and yet reflects the frailties of human nature on the one hand and the ability to learn from experience on the other.

The process of achieving peace in the world is ultimately dependent on people of diverse backgrounds gaining experience in dealing with each other in ways that allow for improvements in life quality while decreasing distrust. Viewing smallpox, polio, AIDS, Guinea worm, onchocerciasis, and measles as common enemies (in the concept of Will Durant as surrogates for an alien invasion) provides the rationale for collaboration rather than division. Accumulating experience in working together for the resolution of common problems not only solves problems but provides an experience base to tackle other problems. The working relationship between people from the U.S.S.R. and the U.S. during the smallpox eradication program was exceptional and certainly made a contribution far beyond the elimination of a disease. Therefore, the eradication of disease may well be an efficient and effective approach to a much larger vision — the promotion of world peace.

SUMMARY

Scientific organization — to determine what is possible, to outline research needs, to organize the appropriate consultation — may be the easiest part of the problem.

Resource development, however, depends on an adequate plan, and it is clear from past experience that for all of the difficulties, money follows the plan. Therefore, the real attention should be on developing a plan that is logical and compelling. Resources will follow. Current interest (including this workshop) demonstrates the utility of the informal scientific network which now exists. The need is to agree on some minimal structure to enhance the network.

An organization to accomplish disease eradication will differ with each problem. It would be counterproductive to attempt an organizational structure to accommodate all future eradication efforts. In fact, it appears that such an organization would stifle innovation for future eradication efforts. Therefore, it appears that an *ad hoc* organization for each eradication effort may provide the most reasonable approach. If this does not turn out to be true, it will always be possible in the future to advocate a formal global organization. However, once such an organization is formed it will never be possible to reverse the process if it is not functional.

Finally, it should be understood that this discussion goes beyond diseases. If eradication efforts are successful, they contribute to the improvement of civilization and especially the necessary experience base that will be required for global peace.

REFERENCES

CDC (Centers for Disease Control and Prevention). 1993. Recommendations of the International Task Force for Disease Eradication. *Morbid. Mortal. Wkly. Rep.* **42(RR–16)**:1–38.

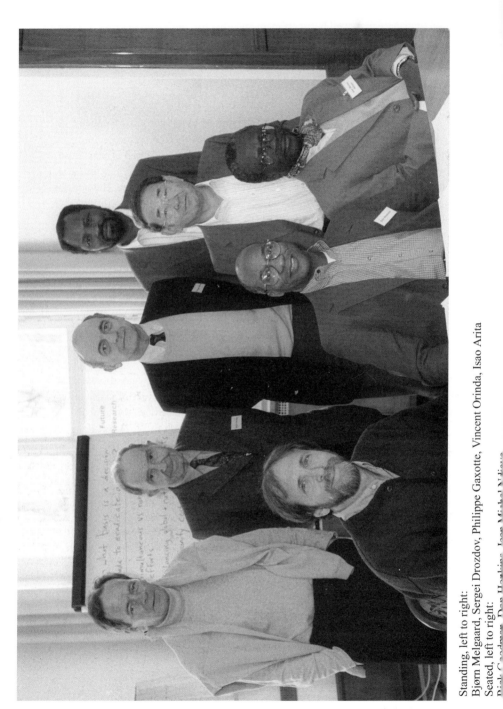

Standing, left to right:
Bjørn Melgaard, Sergei Drozdov, Philippe Gaxotte, Vincent Orinda, Isao Arita
Seated, left to right:
Rick Goodman, Don Hopkins, Jean Michel N'diaye

17

Group Report: When and How Should Eradication Programs Be Implemented?

R.A. GOODMAN, Rapporteur

D.R. HOPKINS, I. ARITA, S.G. DROZDOV,
P. GAXOTTE, B. MELGAARD, J.M. NDIAYE,
V. ORINDA

Where there is no vision, the people perish.
— Ecclesiastes 29:18

INTRODUCTION

Disease eradication programs appear to be conceptually simple: they focus on one clear and unequivocal outcome. At the same time, however, implementation of such programs is extraordinarily difficult because of the unique global and time-driven operational challenges they pose (i.e., they must engage all affected areas without exception, and they require an extremely high level of performance). Previous eradication programs, successful and unsuccessful, have been initiated in many different ways without the benefit of uniform standards based on a thorough review of past experience (CDC 1993; Foege, this volume; Hinman and Hopkins, this volume).

The charge to this group was to address the two fundamental questions of *when* and *how* eradication programs should be implemented. To this end, we identified as a conceptual framework seven steps critical for implementing an eradication program:

1. review and propose potential candidates for eradication;
2. conduct pre-eradication research (e.g., demonstration of elimination);
3. make the decision to eradicate;
4. mobilize resources;
5. conduct strategic planning;

The Eradication of Infectious Diseases
Edited by W.R. Dowdle and D.R. Hopkins © 1998 John Wiley & Sons Ltd.

6. begin and maintain implementation (includes ongoing research); and
7. carry out certification.

The question of "when" a program should be initiated is addressed by steps 1–3, while steps 4–7 address the question of "how" a program should be initiated. For each step, the role of the many participating organizations likely would vary and change.

We have organized this report to address the above framework by examining as major topics: the basis for making a decision to eradicate a disease; mechanisms for decision making; optimizing the relation between eradication programs and ongoing health programs; principles for developing, planning, and implementing eradication programs; estimating and mobilizing resources for eradication; and recommendations, including research priorities. Throughout this chapter, all uses of the term eradication also refer to elimination (cf. Otteson et al., this volume), reflecting the overlap in aims and features of these public health interventions. A particularly important theme of this paper is the critical interaction between disease eradication programs and ongoing health programs.

WHEN SHOULD ERADICATION PROGRAMS BE IMPLEMENTED?

Basis for Making a Decision to Eradicate an Infectious Disease

The decision framework for assessing the potential eradicability of an infectious disease should include three essential categories of criteria: (a) biological/epidemiological criteria; (b) social/political criteria; and (c) the availability or likely availability of adequate economic support.

- First, a candidate disease should satisfy the biological and epidemiological criteria for eradicability (Otteson et al., this volume), which include scientific feasibility; availability of an effective, easily applicable intervention; a capability to readily diagnose infection; and demonstrated elimination of the infection in a large geographic area.

- Second, the social and political criteria to be satisfied include (Hall et al., this volume; Cochi et al., this volume) a substantial and unacceptable burden of disease; a high level of political will and support; shared benefits such that all affected countries are likely to support the effort (if all endemic countries are not supportive, then the eradication program cannot succeed); prediction of a positive benefit/cost ratio within a reasonable time frame; and a general understanding of and agreement to the costs and other consequences of the decision to eradicate. Other political and social considerations include the existence of civil unrest and wars. We concluded that those conditions need not pose insurmountable barriers to disease eradication. For example, the smallpox eradication program succeeded despite civil wars or disturbances in Nigeria, Sudan, Somalia, and West

Bengal/Bangladesh. Other recent examples include cease-fires for polio eradication in Afghanistan and for Guinea worm eradication in Sudan. Addressing such circumstances requires political judgement, negotiating, leadership, and other skills.

- Third, adequate economic support must be available or should be likely to become available. Satisfying this criterion also may take into consideration any potential for synergizing the proposed eradication program with other health efforts, including other eradication programs. For example, the program to eradicate dracunculiasis began as a subgoal of the International Drinking Water Supply and Sanitation Decade (Hopkins 1983), and future prospects include the potential opportunity to synergize the eradication of measles, mumps, and rubella. Eradication programs also offer the potential for enhancing surveillance systems for multiple diseases.

When deciding whether to initiate a global disease eradication campaign, consideration should also be given to the ideal sequencing of different — but potentially concurrent — campaigns. In particular, if two or more global campaigns are to be conducted simultaneously, then it will be important to weigh carefully whether one of the campaigns is near conclusion or is complementary in implementation (e.g., polio and measles), or whether one of the target diseases is already confined to a limited geographic area. The latter situation could accommodate initiation of the regional demonstration of elimination of one disease at the same time a global eradication program for another disease is underway. Examples of this approach include efforts to eliminate measles in the Americas (following the elimination of polio in the Americas) during the global polio eradication campaign, and the expected elimination of dracunculiasis and poliomyelitis almost simultaneously in war-affected areas of southern Sudan.

In addition to the three essential categories of criteria (described above), the decision framework for an eradication program should also take into account certain attributes and potential benefits of eradication, as well as certain limitations, potential risks, and points of caution. Some of the factors (described below) could be classified into both or either categories (potential benefits or potential risks), depending on specific conditions (some of the following are not characteristics only of eradication programs).

The *favorable attributes* and *potential benefits* of eradication programs are that:

- The scope of an eradication program is well-defined, with a clear objective and endpoint.
- The duration of the program is limited.
- The success of the program produces sustainable improvement in health.
- A high benefit/cost ratio is likely.
- The effort is attractive to potential funding sources.
- The program must establish high standards of performance for surveillance, logistics, and administrative support.

- The program develops well-trained and highly motivated health staff.
- The program can assist in the development of health services infrastructure, including, for example, mobilization of endemic communities.
- Equity results because coverage must be extended to all affected areas, including urban, rural, and even remote rural areas.
- The program can provide opportunities for other health benefits (e.g., for dracunculiasis eradication: health education and improved water supply).
- The program can provide opportunities for improved coordination among partners and countries; and
- Efforts may establish dialogue across frontiers of war.

The *limitations, potential risks,* and *points of caution* for eradication programs include:

- Higher short-term costs;
- Increased risk of failure (as a result of the all-or-none construct) and the consequences of failure;
- An inescapable sense of urgency;
- Diversion of attention and resources from equally or more important health problems that are not eradicable, or even others that may be eradicable;
- Detraction or undermining by eradication efforts of the development of general health infrastructure;
- High vulnerability of eradication programs to interruption by war and other civil disturbances;
- Potential that programs will not address national priorities in all countries, and that some countries will not follow the eradication strategy, thereby delaying progress of the global campaign;
- Perception of programs as "donor driven" (this perception also may characterize broader health programs);
- Placement of excessive, counterproductive pressures and demands upon health workers and others; and
- Requirement of special attention for countries with inadequate resources and/or weak health infrastructure (including hit-and-run strategies).

Alternative Mechanisms for Decision Making about Eradication

The prospects for global disease eradication during the 21st century are exciting: several diseases may be considered as potential targets (CDC 1993), underscoring the increased need for a rational, considered approach to selection of diseases and implementation of programs. An examination of previous eradication programs indicates the wide variations in the origins of these programs (Fenner et al., this volume; Foege, this volume; Hinman and Hopkins, this volume). Several proposals for the eradication or elimination of different diseases have been developed as a result of the interests of different combinations of individuals and organizations. In addition, in some instances, early phases were initiated without adequate knowledge, planning, and/or operational research. For example, in the campaign against malaria following the World Health Assembly resolution in 1955, efforts to adjust strategies were introduced too late to ensure success, while the campaign against yaws was never even formally proposed by a World Health Assembly resolution (Hinman and Hopkins, this volume). Smallpox eradication was first proposed by the U.S.S.R. in 1958. The final, intensified smallpox eradication program only began in 1966 when the World Health Assembly adopted a resolution which established a new unit with funding in the World Health Organization (WHO), even though the resolution did not specify a target date. Dracunculiasis "elimination" was proposed in 1986 in a resolution that was followed in 1991 by another World Health Assembly resolution calling for its eradication by 1995. In 1988, the global polio eradication effort began as a result of progress in eliminating polio from the Americas — a regional goal that had been declared in 1985. Measles elimination efforts began in the Western Hemisphere after being stimulated by promising results in many countries in the region; however, global implications for a measles campaign have not yet fully been determined.

A resolution by the World Health Assembly for elimination of neonatal tetanus was adopted in 1989 (target: less than 1 case per district by the year 1996), and leprosy elimination (target: less than 1 case per 10,000 population by the year 2000) was adopted as a goal by the World Health Assembly in 1991. Neither of these latter two resolutions are consistent with the definition of disease elimination that was proposed during this Dahlem Workshop (Otteson et al., this volume).

The group discussed certain perceived limitations in the current mechanisms for investigating, proposing, and selecting candidate diseases for eradication. Some of these issues were highlighted in two of the background papers prepared for this conference (Arita, this volume; Foege, this volume). In considering possible alternative approaches to these processes, we concluded that the pluralism, creativity, and inventiveness that characterize current approaches should be preserved. At the same time, the increasing numbers of potential candidates for eradication warrants a more systematic and coordinated approach in reviewing such candidate diseases. Based on these considerations, we identified three strategic options to improve the critical steps of reviewing proposed candidates for eradication, conducting pre-eradication research, and beginning implementation: (a) continuation of the status quo (Foege, this volume); (b) establishment of a unit at WHO (Arita, this volume); and (c) establishment of an interagency work group. These three options (discussed further below) are neither mutually exclusive nor exhaustive. In addition, different functions and combinations of organizations will be required at different stages of an eradication program. We do not presume to recommend any single option; rather, our purpose is to stimulate further and timely consideration of this important issue.

- *Continuation of status quo*: This option is based on the premise that the role of WHO is necessary, but not sufficient (Foege, this volume). The approach currently involves participation by WHO, some existing task forces, foundations, nongovernmental organizations (NGOs), individuals, and others. It is highly pluralistic and proposals generated in different ways can be formalized by means of a resolution of the World Health Assembly. Potential advantages include pluralism and the capacity for innovation; potential limitations include inadequate coordination and the potential for an overwhelming workload as the number of candidate diseases increases.

- *Establishment of a unit at WHO*: A unit could be established at WHO to analyze, study, and make commitments to eradicating specific diseases. As suggested, the prospects for considering eradication of several diseases over the next two to three decades underscore the need for a systematic and rational approach for obtaining consensus and initiating efforts, and for conducting operational research. This unit would facilitate the submission of proposals to the World Health Assembly for consideration and could provide for the open vetting of proposals. The principal potential advantages to this approach are the systematization of the process and an existing mandate, while potential limitations include bureaucratic impediments and limits on innovation. However, with proper leadership and adequate resources, such impediments might be overcome.

- *Establishment of an interagency work group*: This approach would create a secretariat function outside of WHO and would seek to adapt the best features of the other two alternatives by including multi-sectoral representation (e.g., membership including WHO, donor agencies, private/public sector organizations, and others). Functions would include review of candidate diseases, specification of research needs, and constant dialogue with WHO and all other crucial organizations. Advantages are the capacity for increased dialogue and coordination, and for innovation, while potential limitations include the absence of an existing mandate and the complexity of decision making.

The option of creating a new UN-based agency was also considered; however, this option was not advanced, primarily because of cost and the failure of this option to offer additional advantages over others. A decision to proceed with an eradication program should require a resolution of the World Health Assembly, regardless of the origin of the proposal. Obtaining a resolution by the World Health Assembly is important for ensuring wide commitment and broad input into such decisions by all countries, and to help prevent unwarranted use or trivializing of the concept of eradication. Whatever option is ultimately employed, a paramount consideration is to ensure that high-quality staff are assigned to this important activity.

HOW SHOULD ERADICATION PROGRAMS BE IMPLEMENTED?

Whereas the options outlined above are each intended to ensure that steps 1–3 (see INTRODUCTION) are conducted according to uniform and standard criteria for all candidate diseases, subsequent steps (4–7) will require more pluralism. Thus, the roles of different organizations will evolve during an eradication program.

Historically, one of the most contentious issues regarding eradication programs concerns the relation between such eradication programs and ongoing health programs. Hence, our consideration of how eradication programs should be implemented begins with this topic. It is recognized, however, that more studies and data are needed urgently to better inform and rationalize discussions of this issue.

Optimizing the Relation between Eradication Programs and Ongoing Health Programs

Principles for Optimizing Relations

Three basic principles help to define an approach to optimizing the relation between eradication programs and ongoing health programs (including primary health care) at all levels (community, district, national, regional, and global). First, functioning health systems provide a favorable foundation for eradication programs. Second, communities should not be disrupted by multiple uncoordinated visits or activities for health purposes. Third, with proper planning, eradication programs can indirectly help to strengthen and develop broader health services (Aylward 1997; Tangermann 1997; Taylor Commission 1995). However, the status of primary health care services may vary between countries and within countries, ranging from primary health care programs that work and those that are ineffective, to areas that completely lack such programs. This gradation in availability of primary health care requires that an eradication program be flexible in order to make appropriate use of existing resources (e.g., village-based health workers or health development committees) where health systems are functioning, and to innovate/improvise in settings where health systems are weak or lacking altogether (e.g., by fostering enthusiasm in the population and promoting use of village-based health workers and village development committees). In some locations lacking primary health care, eradication programs may help to establish such capacities and resources. In addition, upon completion of eradication activities in a given locality, eradication-dedicated workers and other resources may be redirected to primary health care or other health programs.

Opportunities for Maximizing/Optimizing Relations by Level

The status of the relation between activities of eradication programs and ongoing programs can be sorted into three categories: (a) those that are synergistic, (b) those that conflict, and (c) those that are neutral. These relations may vary as a function of the level of activity (i.e., community, district, national, regional, and global). The types of major activities include policy, planning/coordination, funding, coordination of donors, training, supervision, monitoring, supply, evaluation, community mobilization, information systems (including surveillance), and health education.

While much attention has been given to the putative or actual "conflict" between eradication activities and ongoing health services, our group emphasized the opportunities for synergy between the two types of programs, at various levels of the health services (Aylward 1997). Some examples include:

1. Community level
    - Promotion of community development committees and community-based health workers (e.g., as in the Guinea worm eradication program)
    - Organization of joint supervisory visits by different programs
    - Concurrent approaches to priority problems for the same target groups
    - Organization of community-based surveillance of local major health problems (e.g., neonatal tetanus and dracunculiasis)
    - Coordination to ensure appropriate spacing/timing of interventions

2. District level
    - Joint planning of complementary and compatible activities by different programs (e.g., the concept of packaging essential health services)
    - To the extent possible, combine or share resources from different programs
    - Use of the same health system to monitor major indicators of each program

3. National level
    - Shared use of functional health management and information system, including mapping (e.g., polio surveillance as part of broader community-based surveillance)
    - Exchange of information (meetings, newsletters)
    - Use of national development plan to reduce conflict/overlap between efforts and ensure balance of human resources
    - Coordination of partners/donors (e.g., polio, dracunculiasis eradication)
    - Use of eradication program as a tool for developing health personnel
    - Adapt/use/emulate selected principles of eradication programs for addressing other selected problems that are not eradicable (e.g., integrated surveillance in AFRO)
    - Mobilization of resources

4. Regional level
    - Sharing of experiences through meetings and program reviews (e.g., dracunculiasis and polio eradication programs)
    - Coordination and monitoring
    - Sharing of laboratory/diagnostic facilities and resources (e.g., polio)
    - Mobilization of resources (e.g., interagency coordinating committees)

5. Global level
    - Assessment of the effect of global trends (e.g., decentralization and priority setting) on eradication
    - Coordination
    - Mobilization of resources

Guiding Principles for Developing, Planning, and Implementing Eradication Programs

Developing Eradication Programs

The decision to undertake a disease eradication program should be based on a combination of biological and epidemiological criteria which take into account the feasibility of eradication, as well as on the social, political, and economic criteria referred to earlier. In addition, the technical interventions should be simple, applicable to all communities (urban and rural), and cost effective.

The target date for eradication (and elimination) programs has particularly crucial implications when compared with other public health initiatives (e.g., control programs, for which there may not be a target date). The target date reflects both the time-limited nature of the eradication program and the discrete outcome, and it underscores the urgency of the effort. Therefore, although the process of establishing a target date should be integrally linked to program planning, the primacy of this step warrants special emphasis. The process of selecting a target date particularly requires a balancing of (a) the availability or likely availability of funding, (b) the attractiveness of certain dates and time lines that are politically opportune to capitalize on organizational interests, and (c) technical feasibility. The duration to the target date should be relatively brief (≤ 10–15 years) — a duration that should be perceived to be finite and realistically achievable. The expected duration of the campaign also relates to budgetary considerations.

To facilitate mobilization of resources, communication strategies must be developed and channels selected for the most effective transmission of technical and other information to critical target groups (e.g., those with political authority [who must support the decision], technicians [who will implement the program] and other health personnel, and communities [who are partners in the effort]). This need includes the requirement of and resources for a communications program with press relations capability at global, regional, and national levels. For example, the World Summit for Children in 1990 helped to mobilize political support for eradication of polio and dracunculiasis. The strongest advocacy points for an eradication program are that it can eliminate a disease forever, it affords a high benefit/cost ratio, and it can be used to strengthen health services. Demonstration of political will and commitment is also essential. Finally, achievement of consensus requires a determination of the different responsibilities at each level (global, regional, and national) and consultation with countries, organizations, and others.

Planning Eradication Programs

Essential steps in planning disease eradication programs include the needs to:

- Conduct a situation analysis of regions and countries by taking into account factors such as the likelihood that other health services will benefit from or be adversely affected by the eradication program, the status of surveillance and health information systems, and the availability of resources;

- Examine and incorporate lessons from past eradication programs;
- Utilize and strengthen existing structures: to the extent possible, eradication programs should use existing structures and systems rather than develop new structures; in addition, eradication programs should not weaken existing primary health care programs;
- Define responsibilities at country, regional, and global levels;
- Learn and obtain input from the private sector (e.g., businesses and NGOs), where relevant;
- Identify requirements for additional operational and epidemiological research; and
- Develop plans of action, including country-specific goals and objectives for implementation plans and a budget.

Implementing Eradication Programs

An overarching principle guiding the implementation of eradication programs is that of maximizing the complementarity of resources devoted to eradication and the efforts of other health programs. While the primary emphasis must be on the disease(s) targeted for eradication, the prevention of other health problems should be simultaneously facilitated whenever possible.

Implementation efforts should, as appropriate, incorporate at least ten additional considerations. First, the approaches and needs specific to different regions, countries, and communities should be recognized and respected (Jamieson 1993). For example, the disease burden itself may be viewed differently among health authorities and by the population. Second, resources should especially be available to assist poorer countries (see next section). Third, efforts should remain flexible and be prepared to respond rapidly to changing circumstances (e.g., polio national immunization days, changes in existing resources, and decreasing population interest as the disease burden decreases). Fourth, logistics, supplies, and monitoring must be adequate, and health workers should be provided with effective supervision, training, regular updates, and feedback. Fifth, a mechanism should be established to share experiences/lessons learned within and across regions, through meetings and other means of communication. Sixth, accurate baseline data and effective surveillance should be assured, enabling the ongoing monitoring of country-by-country progress. Seventh, communications are necessary to maintain motivation of political leaders, and national and external funding sources, as well as to continue providing feedback to health programs and others. Eighth, technical support must be provided to different levels. Ninth, there should be an assurance of the proper mix of technical and management capacity, and the assignment of appropriate responsibility, depending on the phase of program development. Finally, a mechanism should be established to coordinate partners (e.g., international coordinating committees for polio/Expanded Program on Immunization).

Estimating and Mobilizing Resources for Eradication

Categories of need should be determined as early as possible to guide the identification of funds for countries unable to secure sufficient resources on their own. Estimates should be provided that separate internal resource requirements from marginal costs and additional costs. Potential sources of funding may be identified by reviewing previous experiences and approaches, then considering at least three possibilities, including the organization(s) that initiated the eradication program, the potential for "piggybacking" with other initiatives, and donors and organizations that funded the demonstration of elimination of the disease of concern. "Donor mapping" may be used to assist in matching resource needs to the specific interests of potential donors (e.g., interests in laboratory capacity or operational activities).

The solicitation of resources from potential donors can be facilitated by promoting and using the resolution of the World Health Assembly. In addition, a plan of action also should be shared with potential donors, with a reminder that some proportion of resources may be applied to related (but not primarily eradication) activities. Other considerations include: the availability of resources in-country and with the assistance of the private sector; the need to establish a fund for marginal costs for individual countries; recognition that countries with the weakest economies will require the most external assistance; and that proportionately more external assistance will be needed as the eradication program nears completion.

CONCLUSIONS

Disease eradication programs can be distinguished from ongoing health or disease control programs relative to four fundamental factors: the eradication programs' urgency; the requirement for targeted surveillance coupled to a rapid response capability; their requirement of high standards of performance; and their need for a dedicated focal point at the national level. There are varying perceptions and beliefs regarding the relative importance of eradicating a single disease versus attending to other ongoing health needs, including primary health care, and there is a tendency to attribute some problems of primary health care to a diversion of resources and attention by disease eradication efforts. In our assessment of eradication and ongoing programs, eradication was not considered to necessarily be implemented by a completely vertical program. Rather than focusing on a vertical–horizontal dichotomy, we examined approaches to optimizing or creating a complementary relation between an eradication program and ongoing programs at all levels.

Because eradication and ongoing programs constitute potentially complementary approaches to public health, there is need to recognize and address areas of potential overlap, conflict, and synergy. The increase in the number of potentially eradicable diseases underscores the critical importance of phasing and timing, as well as the need for complementarity even among eradication efforts. In addition, eradication has broad ramifications for many sectors (e.g., business, general public) beyond the health sector.

All of these factors increase the need for a more considered, coordinated approach to decision making and preparation for eradication programs.

All eradication programs require some elements of a targeted approach as a consequence of the inherent urgency of eradication and the higher standard of performance that is necessary in an eradication campaign when compared with a control program, or ongoing health services. Nonetheless, potential areas of complementarity include the development of village-based health workers and community development committees, surveillance, health education, and logistical and supervisory support. The problem is not that eradication activities function too well; rather, it is that primary health care activities in many areas do not function well enough. Eradication programs may either impair or strengthen primary health care in some areas. Therefore, efforts are needed to identify and better characterize those factors responsible for the strong functioning of eradication campaigns and to apply them to primary health care. However, where well-functioning primary health care services are available, they should be used as appropriate to facilitate implementation of eradication programs; where primary health care services are not available, eradication programs can and should help to introduce them.

Because of the clear interplay between eradication and other programs, and the consequent sharing of resources, donors should recognize that some proportion of funds may need to be applied to other supportive activities in addition to the eradication effort, per se. Similarly, eradication programs should make use of resources of ongoing programs, whenever possible.

Recommendations and Research Priorities

1. Create an interagency study group to begin as soon as possible to consider what options/approaches are most appropriate for evaluating candidate diseases for eradication.
2. Begin further dialogue and consensus-building to continue refining criteria for disease eradication, as well as the essential steps and principles for implementing eradication programs.
3. Investigate further the impact (both positive and negative effects) of eradication programs on the development of health services infrastructure, and of infrastructure (and lack thereof) on eradication programs.
4. Document the costs of eradication program(s) compared with the benefits, including costs and benefits to both developed and developing countries.
5. To what extent are external resources provided for eradication programs *net* (additive) resources?
6. How can resource mobilization mechanisms and donor coordination for eradication programs be improved (including, for example, the provision of vaccines of adequate quality, and the establishment of global laboratory networks)?
7. Investigate disease surveillance strategies for eradication programs and how to relate those to broader surveillance needs of countries.

8. What aspects of eradication programs can be adapted and usefully applied to implementation of ongoing health services?
9. What communications technologies can be used creatively for the development and implementation of disease eradication programs?

REFERENCES

Aylward, R.B., J. Bilous, R. Tangermann, et al. 1997. Strengthening routine immunization services in the Western Pacific through eradication of poliomyelitis. *J. Infec. Dis.* **175 (Suppl. 1)**:268–271.

CDC (Centers for Disease Control and Prevention). 1993. Recommendations of the International Task Force for Disease Eradication. *Morbid. Mortal. Wkly. Rep.* **42 (RR–16)**:1–38.

Hopkins, D.R. 1983. Dracunculiasis: An eradicable scourge. *Epidemiol. Rev.* **5**:208–219.

Jamieson, D.T., et al., eds. 1993. Disease Control Priorities in Developing Countries. New York. Oxford University Press for the World Bank.

Tangermann, R., M. Costales, and J. Flavier. 1997. Poliomyelitis eradication and its impact on primary health care in the Philippines. *J. Infec. Dis.* **175 (Suppl. 1)**:272–280.

Taylor Commission. 1995. The impact of the Expanded Programme on Immunization and the polio eradication initiative on the health systems in the Americas. Washington, D.C.: Pan American Health Organization.

Author Index

Subject Index

Dahlem Workshop Reports

Forthcoming in 1998

Mechanistic Relationships Between Development and Learning: Beyond Metaphor
Editors: T.J. Carew, R. Menzel & C.J. Shatz
0 471 97702 0   approx 300pp

Titles available

Eradication of Infectious Diseases
Editors: W.R. Dowdle & D.R. Hopkins
0 471 98089 7   220pp   1998

The Evolution of the Universe
Editors: S. Gottlöber & G. Börner
0 471 96524 3   308pp   1997

Saving Our Architectural Heritage: The Conservation of Historic Stone Structures
Editors: N.S. Baer and R. Snethlage
0 471 96526 X   448pp   1997

Regulation of Body Weight: Biological and Behavioral Mechanisms
Editors: C. Bouchard and G.A. Bray
0 471 96373 9   323pp   1996

Upwelling in the Ocean: Modern Processes and Ancient Records
Editors: C.P. Summerhayes, K.-C. Emeis, M.V. Angel. R.L. Smith and B. Zeitzschel
0 471 96041 1   432pp   1995

Aerosol Forcing of Climate
Editors: R.J. Charlson and J. Heintzenberg
0 471 95693 7   432pp   1995

The Role of Nonliving Organic Matter in the Earth's Carbon Cycle
Editors: R.G. Zepp and Ch. Sonntag
0 471 95463 2   350pp   1995

Molecular Aspects of Aging
Editors: K. Esser and G.M. Martin
0 471 95689 9   318pp   1995

Durability and Change: The Science, Responsibility, and Cost of Sustaining Cultural Heritage
Editors: W.E. Krumbein, P. Brimblecombe, D.E. Cosgrove and S. Staniforth
0 471 95221 4   326pp   1994

Acidification of Freshwater Ecosystems: Implications for the Future
Editors: C.E.W. Steinberg and R.F.Wright
0 471 94206 5   420pp   1994

Flexibility and Constraint in Behavioral Systems
Editors: R.J. Greenspan and C.P. Kyriacou
0 471 95252 4   331pp   1994

Cellular and Molecular Mechanisms Underlying Higher Neural Functions
Editors: A.I. Selverston and P. Ascher
0 471 94304 5   344pp   1994

Twins as a Tool of Behavioral Genetics
Editors: T.J. Bouchard, Jr. and P. Propping
0 471 94174 3   326pp   1993

Exploring Brain Functions: Models in Neuroscience
Editors: T.A. Poggio and D.A. Glaser
0 471 93602 2   358pp   1993

Fire in the Environment: The Ecological, Atmospheric, and Climatic Importance of Vegetation Fires
Editors: P.J. Crutzen and J.G. Goldammer
0 471 93604 9   416pp   1993

Global Changes in the Perspective of the Past
Editors: J.A. Eddy and H. Oeschger
0 471 93603 0   400pp   1993

Use and Misuse of the Seafloor
Editors: K.J. Hsü and J. Thiede
0 471 93191 8   456pp   1992

Limiting Greenhouse Effects: Controlling Carbon Dioxide Emissions
Editor: G.I. Pearman
0 471 92945 X   648pp   1992

Ocean Margin Processes in Global Change
Editors: R.F.C. Mantoura, J.-M. Martin and R. Wollast
0 471 92673 6   486pp   1991

Neurodegenerative Disorders: Mechanisms and Prospects for Therapy
Editors: D.L. Price, H. Thoenen and A.J. Aguayo
0 471 92979 4   320pp   1991

Motor Control: Concepts and Issues
Editors: D.R. Humphrey and H.-J. Freund
0 471 92919 0   518pp   1991

Towards a New Pharmacotherapy of Pain
Editors: A.I. Basbaum and J.-M Besson
0 471 92854 2   468pp   1991

Organic Acids in Aquatic Ecosystems
Editors: E.M. Perdue and E.T. Gjessing
0 471 92631 0   360pp   1990

Exchange of Trace Gases between Terrestrial Ecosystems and the Atmosphere
Editors: M.O. Andreae and D.S. Schimel
0 471 92551 9   364pp   1989

Structure and Function of Biofilms
Editors: W.G. Characklis and P.A. Wilderer
0 471 92480 6   404pp   1989

Complex Organismal Functions: Integration and Evolution in Vertebrates
Editors: D.B. Wake and G. Roth
0 471 92375 3   466pp   1989

Etiology of Dementia of Alzheimer's Type
Editors: A.S. Henderson and J.H. Henderson
0 471 92075 4   268pp   1988

Neurobiology of Neocortex
Editors: P. Rakic and W. Singer
0 471 91776 1   474pp   1988

The Changing Atmosphere
Editors: F.S. Rowland and I.S.A. Isaksen
0 471 92047 9   296pp   1988

Biological Perspectives of Schizophrenia
Editors: H. Helmchen and F.A. Henn
0 471 91683 8   368pp   1987

Mechanisms of Cell Injury: Implications for Human Health
Editor: B.A. Fowler
0 471 91629 3   480pp   1987